1989
YEAR BOOK OF
OPHTHALMOLOGY®

# The 1989 Year Book® Series

**Year Book of Anesthesia®:** Drs. Miller, Kirby, Ostheimer, Roizen, and Stoelting

**Year Book of Cardiology®:** Drs. Schlant, Collins, Engle, Frye, Kaplan, and O'Rourke

**Year Book of Critical Care Medicine®:** Drs. Rogers and Parrillo

**Year Book of Dentistry®:** Drs. Rose, Hendler, Johnson, Jordan, Moyers, and Silverman

**Year Book of Dermatology®:** Drs. Sober and Fitzpatrick

**Year Book of Diagnostic Radiology®:** Drs. Bragg, Hendee, Keats, Kirkpatrick, Miller, Osborn, and Thompson

**Year Book of Digestive Diseases®:** Drs. Greenberger and Moody

**Year Book of Drug Therapy®:** Drs. Hollister and Lasagna

**Year Book of Emergency Medicine®:** Dr. Wagner

**Year Book of Endocrinology®:** Drs. Bagdade, Braverman, Halter, Horton, Korenman, Kornel, Metz, Molitch, Morley, Rogol, Ryan, Sherwin, and Vaitukaitis

**Year Book of Family Practice®:** Drs. Rakel, Avant, Driscoll, Prichard, and Smith

**Year Book of Geriatrics and Gerontology:** Drs. Beck, Abrass, Burton, Cummings, Makinodan, and Small

**Year Book of Hand Surgery®:** Drs. Dobyns, Chase, and Amadio

**Year Book of Hematology®:** Drs. Spivak, Bell, Ness, Quesenberry, and Wiernik

**Year Book of Infectious Diseases®:** Drs. Wolff, Barza, Keusch, Klempner, and Snydman

**Year Book of Infertility:** Drs. Mishell, Lobo, and Paulsen

**Year Book of Medicine®:** Drs. Rogers, Des Prez, Cline, Braunwald, Greenberger, Wilson, Epstein, and Malawista

**Year Book of Neonatal and Perinatal Medicine:** Drs. Klaus and Fanaroff

**Year Book of Neurology and Neurosurgery®:** Drs. DeJong, Currier, and Crowell

**Year Book of Nuclear Medicine®:** Drs. Hoffer, Gore, Gottschalk, Sostman, Zaret, and Zubal

**Year Book of Obstetrics and Gynecology®:** Drs. Mishell, Kirschbaum, and Morrow

**Year Book of Oncology:** Drs. Young, Coleman, Longo, Ozols, Simone, and Steele

Year Book of Ophthalmology®: Dr. Laibson

Year Book of Orthopedics®: Dr. Sledge

Year Book of Otolaryngology—Head and Neck Surgery®: Drs. Bailey and Paparella

Year Book of Pathology and Clinical Pathology®: Drs. Brinkhous, Dalldorf, Grisham, Langdell, and McLendon

Year Book of Pediatrics®: Drs. Oski and Stockman

Year Book of Plastic, Reconstructive, and Aesthetic Surgery®: Drs. Miller, Bennett, Haynes, Hoehn, McKinney, and Whitaker

Year Book of Podiatric Medicine and Surgery®: Dr. Jay

Year Book of Psychiatry and Applied Mental Health®: Drs. Talbott, Frances, Freedman, Meltzer, Schowalter, and Weiner

Year Book of Pulmonary Disease®: Drs. Green, Ball, Michael, Peters, Terry, Tockman, and Wise

Year Book of Rehabilitation®: Drs. Kaplan, Frank, Gordon, Lieberman, Magnuson, Molnar, Payton, and Sarno

Year Book of Sports Medicine®: Drs. Shephard, Sutton, and Torg, Col. Anderson, and Mr. George

Year Book of Surgery®: Drs. Schwartz, Jonasson, Peacock, Shires, Spencer, and Thompson

Year Book of Urology®: Drs. Gillenwater and Howards

Year Book of Vascular Surgery®: Drs. Bergan and Yao

**Richard P. Wilson, M.D.**
*Attending Surgeon, Glaucoma Service, Wills Eye Hospital;*
*Associate Professor of Ophthalmology, Jefferson Medical College*
*of Thomas Jefferson University, Philadelphia, Pennsylvania*

1989

# The Year Book of OPHTHALMOLOGY®

Editor-in-Chief
**Peter R. Laibson, M.D.**
Associate Editors
**Raymond E. Adams, M.D.**
**Juan J. Arentsen, M.D.**
**James J. Augsburger, M.D.**
**William E. Benson, M.D.**
**Elisabeth J. Cohen, M.D.**
**Ralph C. Eagle, Jr., M.D.**
**Joseph C. Flanagan, M.D.**
**Leonard B. Nelson, M.D.**
**Robert D. Reinecke, M.D.**
**Robert C. Sergott, M.D.**
**Richard P. Wilson, M.D.**

**Year Book Medical Publishers, Inc.**
**Chicago • London • Boca Raton • Littleton, Mass.**

International Standard Book Number: 0-8151-5265-5

International Standard Serial Number: 0084-392X

Editorial Director, Year Book Publishing: Nancy Gorham
Sponsoring Editor: Gretchen Templeton
Manager, Medical Information Services: Laura J. Shedore
Assistant Director, Manuscript Services: Frances M. Perveiler
Associate Managing Editor, Year Book Editing Services: Elizabeth Griffith
Production Coordinator: Max F. Perez
Proofroom Supervisor: Barbara M. Kelly

# Table of Contents

The material in this volume represents literature reviewed through December 1988.

# Journals Represented

Year Book Medical Publishers subscribes to and surveys almost 850 U.S. and foreign medical and allied health journals. From these journals, the Editors select the articles to be abstracted. Journals represented in this YEAR BOOK are listed below.

Acta Ophthalmolgica
American Journal of Ophthalmology
Annals of Ophthalmology
Archives of General Psychiatry
Archives of Neurology
Archives of Ophthalmology
Binocular Vision
British Journal of Ophthalmology
British Journal of Plastic Surgery
British Journal of Radiology
Canadian Journal of Ophthalmology
Cancer
Cornea
International Ophthalmology Clinics
Investigative Ophthalmology and Visual Science
Japanese Journal of Ophthalmology
Journal of the American Medical Association
Journal of Cataract and Refractive Surgery
Journal of Neurology, Neurosurgery and Psychiatry
Journal of Pediatric Ophthalmology and Strabismus
Journal of Refractive Surgery
Klinische Monatsblatter fur Augenheilkunde
Mayo Clinic Proceedings
Medical Journal of Australia
Neurology
New England Journal of Medicine
Ophthalmic Research
Ophthalmic Surgery
Ophthalmologica
Ophthalmology
Orbit
Retina Journal of Retinal and Vitreous Diseases
Survey of Ophthalmology

# Publisher's Preface

We are delighted to welcome Peter R. Laibson, M.D., and his associates, Raymond E. Adams, M.D., Juan J. Arentsen, M.D., James J. Augsburger, M.D., William E. Benson, M.D., Elisabeth J. Cohen, M.D., Ralph C. Eagle, Jr., M.D., Joseph C. Flanagan, M.D., Leonard B. Nelson, M.D., Robert D. Reinecke, M.D., Robert C. Sergott, M.D., and Richard P. Wilson, M.D., as editors of the YEAR BOOK OF OPHTHALMOLOGY.

This team is carrying on the tradition of distinguished editorial direction for the YEAR BOOK commencing with this 1989 edition. We congratulate them and extend our appreciation for their superb work.

# Introduction

This first issue of the YEAR BOOK OF OPHTHALMOLOGY from Wills Eye Hospital has each specialty chapter introduced by a special article written by the Associate Editor in charge of that section. These introductory sections are worthwhile reading, as they highlight what each Associate Editor believes is important in his or her field for the year. For example, Dr. Augsburger writes on the randomized clinical trial for patients with choroidal and ciliary body melanomas, Dr. Benson writes on postsurgical endophthalmitis, and Dr. Eagle discusses the genetics of retinoblastoma.

Several Associate Editors have gone somewhat afield and written on socioeconomic topics, such as Dr. Reinecke on the Hsiao Report concerning resource-based relative value scales. It is essential that every ophthalmologist know about the Hsiao Report and how it may affect their practice.

Dr. Sergott has described an ophthalmic subspecialty in transition in his review of neuro-ophthalmology. It may become more of a surgical subspecialty with procedures such as optic nerve decompression. Other Associate Editors review their specific fields with a look to the future, particularly Dr. Flanagan discussing use of the contact laser in oculoplastic surgery. The wide variety of new developments in all of ophthalmology makes it almost impossible for any single editor or even several editors to cover the entire field satisfactorily. The YEAR BOOK OF OPHTHALMOLOGY, now edited at Wills Eye Hospital, hopes to provide you with a broad view of general and specialty ophthalmology, selecting from the past what is considered important for the present and speculating what may be useful or necessary in the future. Our expanding field is becoming more and more difficult to grasp, but through this YEAR BOOK, we hope to provide a useful synopsis of the current literature as well as a glimpse of the future.

Peter R. Laibson, M.D.

# 1 Cataract

---

## Cataract Review: 1988

RAYMOND E. ADAMS, M.D.
*Cherry Hill, New Jersey*

The following highlights of 1988 will be discussed in this introduction: continuous capsulotomy; water-assisted cataract removal; posterior chamber intraocular lenses; the aging eye; cataract formation; and the Snellen visual acuity test. We also relate a fairy story.

### Continuous Capsulotomy

The popular can-opener capsulotomy opening evolved from the Kelman Christmas tree and earlier primitive techniques. These were fairly safe, simple, and effective procedures but not problem free. The Neuhann Capsulorhexis (1) technique allows for a continuous, circular opening in the anterior lens capsule. This has an advantage only in phacoemulsification, not in planned extracapsular cataract extraction. After the lens is emulsified, the smooth circular edge of the anterior capsule provides controlled in-the-bag intraocular lens implantation and a lessened postoperative likelihood that the haptic will slide out of the bag. Also, a capsulorhexis opening lacks multiple tears, which can extend to the posterior capsule during hydrodissection or manipulation.

During phacoemulsification the smaller continuous anterior capsule opening may protect the corneal endothelium by shielding the cornea from direct ultrasonic activity or lens fragments. Phacoemulsification combined with a small capsulotomy opening is nicknamed endocapsular or intercapsular phacoemulsification.

Capsulorhexis is challenging to learn and cannot always be completed. Success is dependent on the elasticity and thickness of the anterior capsule. Finesse with a bent 25-gauge needle or fine-toothed forceps may be required. Nevertheless, this is a good technique and I recommend it. Be prepared to convert to the can-opener capsulotomy when the capsule rips out of control.

### Water-Assisted Cataract Removal

Separation of splitting of the lens structure with water is called hydrolamellar dissection. The capsule, cortex, or nucleus separates by this simple procedure. Briefly, after performing the capsulotomy, saline is forced under the anterior capsule with a 2-ml syringe and a 30-gauge cannula. The result is a splitting of the posterior tissue planes. Some envision this to be a "cushioning nest" of posterior cortex. This is turn covers and protects the posterior capsule during phaco or planned extracapsular extraction (2).

Hydrodissection also loosens the more dense lens tissue to permit lens rotation for emulsification or lifting the lens edge out of the capsular bag. This practice may prevent one of the most grave complications of cataract extraction (posterior capsule rupture with loss of the nucleus into the vitreous cavity).

London's Moorfield's Hospital has used hydrodissection for planned extracapsular cataract extraction. I routinely use hydrolamellar dissection before phaco and find it helpful in most types of cataracts. However, be careful not to use excessive force. This can result in blow-out of the lens or extensive splitting of the capsule.

## Posterior Chamber Intraocular Lens Without Capsular or Zonular Support

Intraocular lens (IOL) suturing resurfaced in 1988 (3). Aphakic patients with torn or missing capsules or zones may have the IOL sutured to the sclera in the ciliary sulcus with nonadsorbable 10−0 Prolene. This technique was carried out in six patients in whom contact lenses failed and anterior chamber IOLs were countraindicated.

The potential risks of this procedure are intraoperative hemorrhage, permanent scleral fistulas, vitreous disturbance after anterior vitrectomy with cystoid macular edema or retinal detachment, difficulty in assuring the exact placement of the haptics, calculation of the lens power as related to lens position, tilting or rotation of the optic inducing astigmatism or altering the effective lens power, and knot slippage leading to subluxation or dislocation.

The potential problems of sutured ciliary sulcus IOLs must be compared to parallel complications with anterior chamber IOLs. Anterior chamber lenses have a higher incidence and great variety of complications compared with the standard in-the-bag posterior chamber lens.

Using the suturing technique, a small group of successful posterior chamber implantations has been carried out in aphakic patients when combined with corneal transplantation, anterior segment reconstruction, and postlensectomy/vitrectomy.

## The Aging Eye

Results of Olbert's (4) study clearly indicate a relatively steady decrease in anterior chamber depth from age 30 on, with a corresponding increase in lens thickness. In women the anterior chamber depth as measured from the anterior surface of the lens was 0.19 mm smaller than that in men.

Patients with acute angle-closure glaucoma have very shallow or absent anterior chambers (5). Yearly examination of the anterior chamber depth and lens thickness is recommended in all potential high-risk patients. Hypermetropic patients and elderly women appear more frequently to have angle-closure glaucoma.

Annual echographic examination (A-scan) of the lens thickness and anterior chamber depth can be used to predict impending acute angle-closure glaucoma. Preventive measures can then be brought into play before an attack occurs.

Another question is whether the eye shortens with old age. Fledelius concurs that, with increasing age, lens thickness increases and the anterior chamber depth decreases, but he favors eye size stability in old age (5).

## Cataract Formation

The human lens has been likened to a "biologic dosimeter for radiation exposure in situ" (6). Attempts to relate cataract formation with various metabolic, external, or other means has always interested ophthalmologists. In this age of preventive medicine, the prevention of cataract formation and/or the dissemination of information to patients takes on medical, moral, and legal ramifications.

Exposure to sunlight or ultraviolet radiation has been suggested as a cause of cataract formation. Strongly supporting this theory is the work of Taylor et al. (7), who report on Chesapeake Bay watermen and cataract development. This group found "a clear association between the degree of ultraviolet B exposure and the risk of cortical cataracts. The subjects with cortical cataracts had a greater exposure to ultraviolet radiation from the age of 16 on than those without cortical cataracts." A 3.3-fold increased risk for cortical cataracts was observed in the group exposed to ultraviolet B, but no association was found with nuclear cataracts or between ultraviolet A exposure and nuclear or cortical cataracts.

Ultraviolet A (400–320 nm) induces sun tanning, whereas ultraviolet B (320–290 nm) causes sunburn, blistering, and skin cancer; ultraviolet C (290–100 nm) does not penetrate the earth's surface (8).

Taylor et al.'s conclusions based upon their observation of the Chesapeake Bay watermen were that "it is prudent to protect the eyes from unnecessary exposure to the ultraviolt B" (7). Ultraviolet energy varies markedly during the day and is highest in the summer between 10 AM and 2 PM. Exposure can be reduced ("half") by simply wearing a hat with a brim and ("5%") ordinary sunglasses; however, a set of close-fitting ultraviolet-absorbing lenses gives maximal protection.

Microwave and ionizing radiation (9) most commonly causes anterior or posterior subcapsular lenticular opacities. This may be related to the deformation of heat-labile enzymes (such as glutathone peroxide) or thermoelastic expansion, through which pressure waves in the aqueous humour cause direct physical damage to the lens cells. Ionizing radiation (x-irradiation and gamma rays) usually cause the posterior subcapsular cataract.

Various vitamins are thought to influence the antioxidant status and reduce the risk of cataract formation. They are vitamin C, vitamin E, and the carotenoids. The hypothesis is that the lens antioxidant defense may play a role in cataractogenesis (10).

The calcium content of the lens and its possible imbalance in cataract development has been studied for decades. There appears to be a marked increase in calcium in mature cataracts. However, diseases characterized by prolonged hypocalcemia may induce cataract development over time. An example is primary hypoparathyroidism. Unexpectedly, the cataract patients had an increased aqueous humor concentration of magnesium relative to the serum concentration (11).

Cataract development was investigated in an HMO population who were considered to be more health conscious and less apt to smoke cigarettes. Cataractogenic considerations included diabetes mellitus, ocular trauma, roentgen ray irradiation, ultraviolet light, myopia, and corticosteroid therapy, as well as nutrition and family history. However, the conclusion was that the influence of these factors is poorly understood and may sometimes be challenged (12). In this series, 50% of the study group had sustained blunt trauma, or used steroids or had inflammation or diabetes mellitus. The latter patient was 3.5 years older than the nondiabetics at the time of cataract extraction.

## A Fairy Story

Each year health care providers are under greater review by powerful federal regulatory agencies in an attempt to ensure compliance with established Medicare guidelines. Donald M. Berwick, M.D. (13) contrasts this problem to industry:

"Imagine two assembly lines, monitored by two foremen.

"Foreman 1 walks the line, watching carefully. 'I can see you all,' he warns. 'I have the means to measure your work, and I will do so. I will find those among you who are unprepared or unwilling to do your jobs, and when I do there will be consequences. There are many workers available for these jobs, and you can be replaced.'

"Foreman 2 walks a different line, and he too watches. 'I am here to help you if I can,' he says. 'We are in this together for the long haul. You and I have a common interest in a job well done. I know that most of you are trying very hard, but sometimes things can go wrong. My job is to notice opportunities for improvement—skills that could be shared, lessons from the past, or experiments to try together—and to give you the means to do your work even better than you do now. I want to help the average ones among you, not just the exceptional few at either end of the spectrum of competence.'

"Which line works better? Which is more likely to do the job well in the long run? Where would you rather work?"

Foreman 1 relies on inspection to improve quality because quality is best achieved by discovering "bad apples" and removing them from the work force through "recertification," "deterrence" through litigation, and the search for "outliers"—". . . statistics far enough from the average that chance alone is unlikely to provide a good excuse." This game is not fun, and the workers are afraid and angry.

"The Japanese learned first—from American theorists, ironically— that there were far better ways to improve quality, and the result is international economic history." Nevertheless, in 1988, ophthalmology responded to "Foreman 1" with added instrumentation to prove that we are not the "bad apple"! Paul P. Lichter (14) writes, "I am concerned that when we devise some form of test with a numeric value to substitute for our clinical judgment, we open the door to bureaucratic decision on whether or not cataract surgery is justified." The use of the lens opacity meter, contrast sensitivity devices, and glare tests are such examples.

## Snellen Is Out, Sine Wave Is In

The Snellen visual acuity test is a less standardized test than once believed. Letter charts pose perceptual difficulties (different letters, i.e., "L" vs. the "E"), and the number of letters per line (crowding phenomenon), luminance, and patient literary or cognition skills influence test results. Arthur P. Ginsburg, PhD (15) explains that the use of the Snellen visual acuity test is based on historical precedent as there is "little or no functional relationship between Snellen acuity and everyday visual performance."

The use of sine wave gratings can overcome the limitations of the Snellen visual acuity test and are the most sensitive visual targets, being easier to administer than low-contrast letter tests. Audiologists learned that pure tones are the best targets with which to test hearing.

Neumann et al. (16) studied 78 patients using a Snellen eye chart outdoors in the central Florida mid-summer sunlight. Of the cataractous eyes, almost 70% had visual acuities of at least 2 Snellen lines worse when measured outdoors. The investigators concluded, "It is clear that indoor Snellen visual acuity cannot be used as the sole criterion for visual impairment. Cataract patients often present with complaints of disabling glare yet have good visual acuities when tested outdoors."

When the illumination of the Snellen chart was controlled with a light meter and a 1.5-mm pin-hole to control pupil size, Marmor Gawande (17) found that modest refractive degradation of acuity in normal persons results in a broad loss of contrast sensitivity.

Sjöstrand and Hard (18) stated that the major effect of glare in cataract patients is the contrast-lowering effect and is weakly correlated with Snellen visual acuity. Zulauf and Flammer (19) suggested that visual tests use green color and horizontally oriented gratings. Blanchard (20) uses Vistech charts for distant and near-vision testing as ". . . it rivals the sensitivity of single (intraocular) pressure measurements in selecting those at risk for glaucoma." The use of these charts for health screening fairs was recommended.

In 1988 ophthalmology responded to the federal regulators' demand for documentation of visual loss in cataract. The result is the emergence of new technology to appease the government and at the same time offer advancement of visual testing.

*References*

1. Haefliger E, Neuhann T: The Neuhann capsulorhexis: A safe technique for all-in-the-bag implantation. *Klin Monatsbl Augenheilkd* 192:435–438, 1988.

2. Bailley WR: Phacoemulsification in the nest: A new technique to protect the posterior capsule. *Phaco & Foldables* 1:1–4, 1988.
3. Hu BV, Shin DM, Gibbs KA, et al: Implantation of posterior chamber lens in the absence of capsular and zonular support. *Arch Ophthalmol* 106:416–420, 1988.
4. Olbert D: Relation of the depth of the anterior chamber to the lens thickness: Clinical significance. *Ophthalmol Res* 20:149–153, 1988.
5. Fledelius HC: Refraction and eye size in the elderly. *Acta Ophthalmol* 66:241–248, 1988.
6. Worgul BV: Accelerated heavy particles and the lens. *Ophthalmol Res* 20:143–148, 1988.
7. Taylor HR, West SK, Rosenthal FS, et al: Effect of ultraviolet radiation on cataract formation. *N Engl J Med* 319:1429–1433, 1988.
8. Söderberg PG: Acute cataract in the rat after exposure to radiation in the 300 nm wavelength region. *Acta Ophthalmol* 66:141–152, 1988.
9. Lipman RM, Tripathi BJ, Tripathi RC: Cataracts induced by microwave and ionizing radiation. *Surv Ophthalmol* 33:200–210, 1988.
10. Jacques PF, Chylach LT Jr, McGandy RB, et al: Antioxidant status in persons with and without senile cataract. *Arch Ophthalmol* 106:337–340, 1988.
11. Ringvold A, Sagen E, Bjerve KS, et al: The calcium and magnesium content of the human lens and aqueous humour. *Acta Ophthalmol* 66:153–156, 1988.
12. Schwab L: Cataract extraction: Risk factors in a health maintenance organization under 60 years of age. *Arch Ophthalmol* 66:1062–1066, 1988.
13. Berwick DM: Continuous improvement as an ideal in health care. *N Engl J Med* 320:53–56, 1989.
14. Lichter PP: Interpreting tests-implications for cataract surgery (editorial). *Ophthalmology* 95:1–2, 1988.
15. Ginsburg A: Need for standard glare, contrast sensitivity tests. *Ocular Surgery News*, March 15, 1988, pp 25–31.
16. Neumann AC, McCarty GR, Steedle TO, et al: The relationship between indoor and outdoor Snellen visual acuity in cataract patients. *J Cataract Refract Surg* 14:35–39, 1988.
17. Marmor MF, Gawande A: Effect of visual blur on contrast sensitivity: Clinical implications. *Ophthalmology* 95:139–143, 1988.
18. Sjöstrand J, Abrahamsson M, Hård A: Glare disability as a cause of deterioration of vision in cataract patients. *Acta Ophthalmol* (Copenh) 65:103–106, 1987.
19. Zulauf M, Flammer J, Signer C: Spatial brightness contrast sensitivity measured with white, green, red and blue light. *Ophthalmologia* 196:43–48, 1988.
20. Blanchard D: Contrast sensitivity: A useful tool in glaucoma. *Glaucoma* 10:151–153, 1988.

**Effect of Ultraviolet Radiation on Cataract Formation**

Taylor HR, West SK, Rosenthal FS, Muñoz B, Newland HS, Abbey H, Emmett EA (Johns Hopkins Univ)
*N Engl J Med* 319:1429–1433, Dec 1, 1988

There are photobiologic and biochemical reasons why exposure to sunlight may cause senile cataracts, but firm epidemiologic evidence is lacking. The occurrence of cataract was related to levels of annual ocular exposure of 838 watermen (mean age, 53 years) from age 16. Exposure was calculated from the occupational history and laboratory and field measurements of solar exposure. All worked on Chesapeake Bay.

The median annual ocular exposure was 0.02 Maryland sun year (the maximum of 0.09 would represent work on the water all day each day of the year without a hat or glasses). Thirteen percent of the men had some cortical lens opacity and 27% had some nuclear opacity. Ultraviolet B (UBV) exposure was significantly greater than expected for watermen with cortical opacities. For those with cortical opacities excess exposure occurred annually after age 15 years. Those whose annual average exposure was in the upper quartile had a relative risk of cortical cataract of 3.3.

A clear relationship between UVB exposure and the risk of cortical cataract was evident in this study of watermen. No such association was found for nuclear cataract or for UVA exposure. Experimentally, the lens is most vulnerable to radiation in the UVB band, and it would seem wise to avoid unnecessary exposure to UVB. In addition to wearing sunglasses with UBV-absorbing lenses at times of peak exposure, a hat with a brim is helpful.

---

**The Neuhann Capsulorhexis: A Safe Technique for All-in-the-Bag Implantation**
Haefliger E, Neuhann Th (Kantonsspitals Liestal, München; Krankenanstalt Rotes Kreuz, Munich, West Germany)
*Klin Monatsbl Augenheilkd* 192:435–438, 1988                    1–2

---

Previous histologic studies of pseudophakic cadaver eyes have shown poor correlation between the actual postoperative position of anterior lens capsule openings and those intended intraoperatively by the surgeon. It has been suggested that the position of the lens capsule opening may be an important factor in the outcome of intraocular lens implantation. However, this assumption has been difficult to prove because of the great variation in postoperative lens capsule opening positions. Moreover, this variability makes it impossible to demontrate the advantages of all-in-the-bag lens implantation over sulcus fixation.

With conventional techniques, the stability of the peripheral edge of the anterior lens capsule is lost after excavation of the lens material. The Neuhann capsulorhexis creates a continuous circular opening in the anterior lens capsule that provides maximum stability in the zonulolenticular diaphragm, even after the lens material has been excavated, thus facilitating control of the lens haptic for in-the-bag implantation. Capsulorhexis reduces the morphological variability of the anterior capsule and allows easy confirmation of the position of the lens opening both during and after operation. A more uniform position of lens loops will enable a more

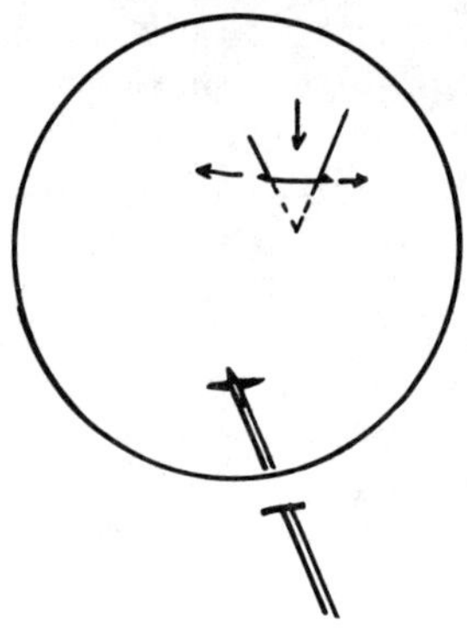

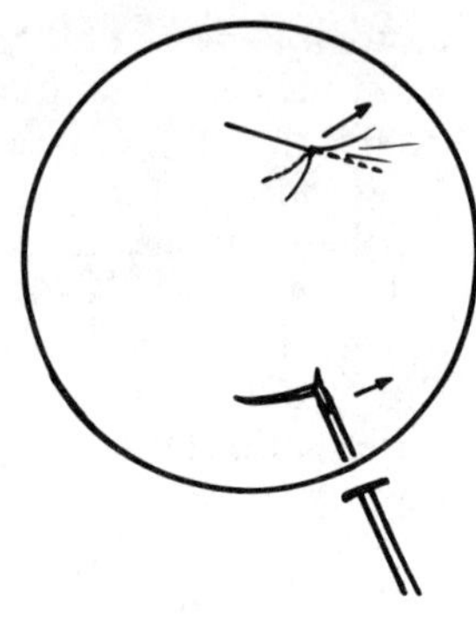

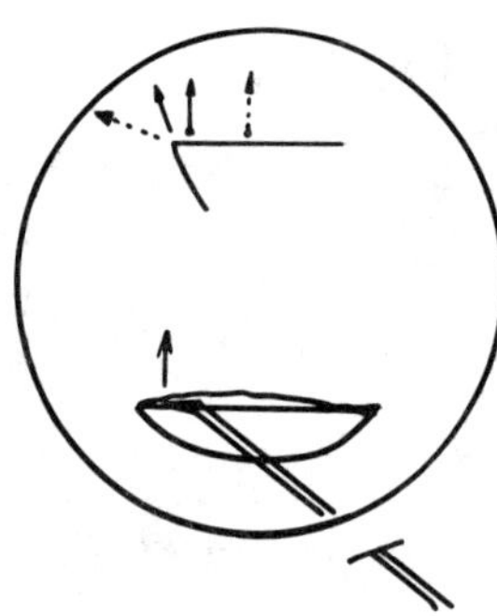

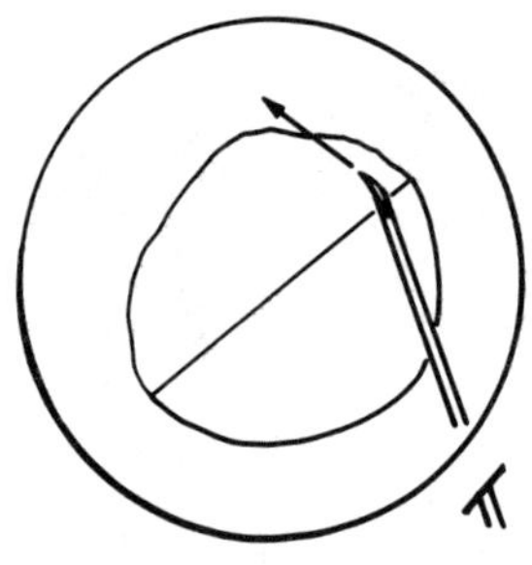

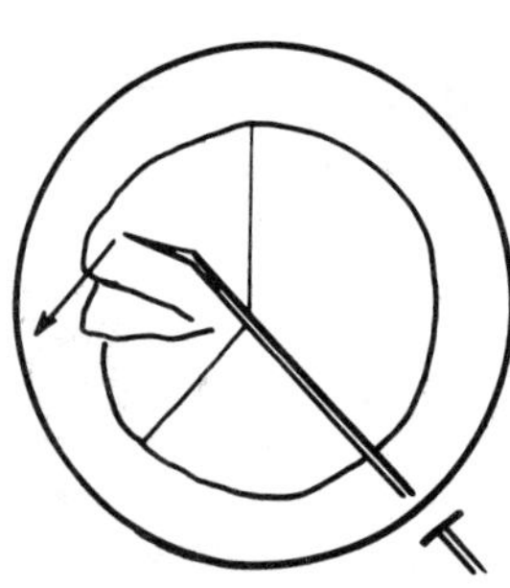

**Fig 1–1 (upper left).**—The point of a burr-free needle is inserted through the anterior lens capsule about 3 mm from the center. The diagram demonstrates the vectorial forces required to obtain a linear cut without creating a radial cut.

**Fig 1–2 (upper right).**—The linear incision is extended by lifting the lens capsule, using a tenting motion, with the sharp side of the needle facing upward from underneath the lens capsule.

**Fig 1–3 (center left).**—As soon as the central part of the lens capsule starts to camber, the capsule can be torn by pushing (the needle) forward along the periphery of the camber. In the diagram, the *dotted line* indicates the radial tear that will occur if the point of the needle is inserted too close to the center.

**Fig 1–4 (center right).**—The capsule tear is guided through the vector field created by the cambering central portion of the lens capsule.

**Fig 1–5 (lower left).**—The lens capsule is torn along the lower circumference of the camber. Toward the end of the tear trajectory, the point of the needle usually needs to be repositioned several times.

(Courtesy of Haefliger E, Neuhann Th: *Klin Monatsbl Augenheilkd* 192:435–438, 1988.)

valid comparison between various available techniques of intraocular lens implantation.

Instructions for performing the Neuhann capsulorhexis and an explanation of the mechanical principles on which it is based are given in Figures 1–1 through 1–5. The technique is as follows:

*Technique.*—The point of a burr-free needle is inserted through the anterior lens capsule about 3 mm from the center. The diagram (Fig 1–1) demonstrates the vectorial forces required to obtain a linear cut without creating a radial cut. The linear incision is extended by lifting the lens capsule using a tenting motion, with the sharp side of the needle facing upward from underneath the lens capsule (Fig 1–2). As soon as the central part of the lens capsule starts to camber, the capsule can be torn by pushing (the needle) forward along the periphery of the camber. In Figure 1–3, the *dotted line* indicates the radial tear that will occur if the point of the needle is inserted too close to the center. The capsule tear is guided through the vector field created by the cambering central portion of the lens capsule (Fig 1–4). The lens capsule tear is continued along the lower circumference of the camber (Fig 1–5). Toward the end of the tear's trajectory, the point of the needle usually needs to be repositioned several times.

▶ With this technique a more circular anterior capsular lens opening may be facilitated, which should allow better haptic placement in the sac. The surgery appears simple in the diagrams, but this is not always the case. It is worthwhile, however, to try this procedure.— P.E. Adams, M.D.

---

**Retinal Phototoxicity From the Operating Microscope: The Role of Inspired Oxygen**
Jaffe GJ, Irvine AR, Wood IS, Severinghaus JW, Pino GR, Haugen C (Univ of California, San Francisco)
*Ophthalmology* 95:1130–1141, August 1988                     1–3

---

The threshold exposure duration for producing photic retinal damage depends on many factors, including wavelength and intensity of the incident light, and body temperature. Arterial oxygen tension $(PaO_2)$ may also be important. Light-induced damage from an operating microscope may be potentiated by excess inspired oxygen provided during general anesthesia or via nasal cannula during local anesthesia. Experiments were conducted to determine if retinal damage produced by the light source of the operating microscope is related to inspired oxygen concentration $(FiO_2)$.

Phakic rhesus monkeys were used. One eye of each animal was exposed to light under conditions of 99% $FiO_2$ and the other was exposed under 21% $O_2$. Three of 4 locations on each retina were exposed to light for durations of 1½ to 20 minutes per exposure. Fundus photographs and fluorescein angiograms were obtained 24–72 hours after exposure. Retinal phototoxic lesions were produced after an average of 5 minutes of light exposure under 21% and 99% $O_2$. Oxygen potentiated the light damage clinically and histologically. In both conditions, lesion size was directly related to the duration of light exposure. Lesions near threshold produced with 99% $FiO_2$ were 1.6–6.1 times larger than the corresponding lesions formed with 21% $FiO_2$. Histologic damage was more severe in lesions produced under high $O_2$ conditions. Retinal repair occurred in lesions produced under both high and low $O_2$ conditions. Photoreceptor regeneration was almost complete by 18 weeks, whereas retinal pigment epithelial recovery took at least 22 weeks.

These findings have important implications for clinical practice. The operating microscope can produce retinal photoxicity rapidly, and $O_2$ given during ophthalmic procedures can potentiate the damage if appropriate precautions are not taken.

▶ The slow surgeon using an operatory microscope may endanger ocular tissues in several ways. These may include lengthy ocular hypotension triggering expulsive choroidal hemmorhage, prolonged irrigation with "balanced" saline solution producing corneal endothelial damage, and extended opening of the wound increasing exposure to infection.—R.E. Adams, M.D.

---

**Nd:YAG Laser Shock Waves in Artificial Eyes**
Wilmanns I, Stodtmeister R, Pillunat LE (Univ Eye Hosp Bonn, Bonn-Venusberg; Univ Eye Hosp Ulm, Ulm, West Germany)
*Ophthalmologica* 196:210–215, 1988                                           1–4

---

Laser pulses cause breakdown of material because large amounts of energy are concentrated in a very small volume. However, optical breakdown in the eye is accompanied by destructive mechanical effects caused by phase changes and shock waves. The shock waves are not restricted to the point of origin but expand throughout the eye. They also strike healthy structures. The shock waves can be felt even at the back of a patient's head during treatment. Shock wave amplitudes produced by single and multiple pulses of 1.064 μm Nd:YAG laser energy in artificial eyes of various lengths were measured.

As the laser pulse energy was increased the shock waves of higher amplitudes appeared 0.1 msec later for a single pulse than for a pulse sequence. The effects observed were not caused by mechanical resonance. Peak pulse amplitudes in the artificial eyes of different length were found to increase linearly as a function of the energy transferred into the eye. The peak amplitudes of pulse sequences were only half of those for single pulses of comparable energy. In laser surgery these sequences may be preferable if they achieve the same effect.

The recorded waveforms of shock waves in artificial eyes of different lengths are not caused by reflections or resonances. All curves were found to be similar. Their peak amplitudes appeared after the first millisecond and decreased rapidly afterward. The visible effects of optically induced breakdown in solid material have previously been shown to differ from those in water, but no differences in the shock wave patterns in the 2 media were found in this study. Peak pulse amplitudes in artificial eyes of different lengths increased linearly as a function of the energy transferred into the eyes.

▶ The incidence of retinal detachment has declined with the shift to extracapsular cataract surgery. To maintain this impressive trend, posterior capsulotomies should be performed when capsule opacification requires laser energy of less than 2.0 mJ, at least in the experimental situation.—R.E. Adams, M.D.

---

**Use of Photographic Techniques to Grade Nuclear Cataracts**
West SK, Rosenthal F, Newland HS, Taylor HR (Johns Hopkins Univ)
*Invest Ophthal Vis Sci* 29:73–77, January 1988                    1–5

---

Photographing cataracts allows for documenting lens opacities objectively and grading them using expert graders or densitometric analysis. The feasibility and reliability of 2 photographic methods of grading nuclear opacities were examined. Forty-one eyes were photographed using a regular Topcon SL-5D photo slit-lamp and a Topcon SL-45 camera. The photos were graded against a set of 4 standard photographs of increasing nuclear opacification, and densitometric analysis was done on both sets.

Agreement between the results of clinical slit-lamp examination and gradings of photos was only fair. Interobserver reliability was high with photos taken using the photo slit-lamp, and the severity grading of these photos correlated well with densitometric analyses.

Photodocumentation of nuclear opacities seem feasible. The photo slit-lamp is much more reliable and reproducible than clinical examination is, particularly when the latter relies on a written description. Epidemiologic field surveys of cataracts can use photographs of the lens nucleus obtained by photo slit-lamp and a standard set of photographs of nuclear opacity.

▶ Cataract grading is simple yet difficult to document clinically. Slit-lamp photodocumentation is accurate and has reliable interobserver grading. Photography offers a means of grading cataracts in office, clinic, or epidemiologic surveys.—R.E. Adams, M.D.

---

**The Relationship Between Indoor and Outdoor Snellen Visual Acuity in Cataract Patients**
Neumann AC, McCarty GR, Steedle TO, Sanders DR, Raanan MG (Neumann Eye Inst, DeLand, Fla; Chicago)
*J Cataract Refract Surg* 14:35–39, January 1988                    1–6

---

Glare may be described as a contrast-lowering effect of light that enters the eye so as to inhibit distinct vision. Light is scattered in the eye by opacities in the lens, vitreous, or other clear media. The authors compared Snellen visual acuities as measured indoors and outdoors in 78 patients with 106 cataractous eyes.

About three fourths of cataractous eyes had Snellen acuities of 20/40 or better when tested indoors, whereas fewer had one third had acuities this good when tested outdoors facing the sun. Three eyes (2.8%) had acuity worse than 20/80 indoors compared with 29.2% when tested outdoors. Ten eyes had outdoor acuities worse than 20/200. More than two thirds of eyes had outdoor acuities at least 2 Snellen lines worse than indoor values. The median difference between indoor and outdoor acuity was 3 Snellen lines (table).

Indoor Snellen acuity should not be the sole criterion for visual impairment in cataract patients, who often complain of disabling glare but have good indoor acuity.

Glare testing may be used to ascertain the need for surgery. Both the Miller-Nadler glare tester and the brightness acuity tester were developed using actual outdoor vision testing of cataract patients.

Summary of Snellen Line Differences in Indoor and Outdoor Best Corrected Visual Acuity

| | Number of Snellen Lines* | | |
| Cataract Type | Number | Median | Range |
| --- | --- | --- | --- |
| Pure nuclear sclerosis | 30 | 2 | −3 to 6 |
| Nuclear sclerosis + posterior subcapsular opacities | 41 | 3 | 0 to 8 |
| Other cataractous combinations | 35 | 3 | −2 to 7 |
| All eyes | 106 | 3 | −3 to 8 |

*Negative values indicate that visual acuity was better when measured outdoors. Positive values indicate decreases in visual acuity when measured outdoors.

(Courtesy of Neumann AC, McCarty GR, Steedle TO, et al: *J Cataract Refract Surg* 14:35–39, January 1988.)

▶ When is the patient ready for cataract surgery, and when is surgery justified? Cataract assessment in the office may not correlate with the patient's functional visual impairment, which interferes with occupation or life-style. The authors use an objective method to compare indoor vision and outdoor vision with glare disability to justify the need for cataract surgery.—R.E. Adams, M.D.

## Comparison of the SRK II Formula and Other Second Generation Formulas

Sanders DR, Retzlaff J, Kraff MC (Univ of Illinois, Chicago; Medford, Ore)
*J Cataract Refract Surg* 14:136–141, March 1988
1–7

The SRK power formula has become the most widely used means of calculating implant power. It is, at worst, clinically equivalent in accuracy to earlier theoretic formulas based on the application of geometric optics to schematic eye models. A modified SRK formula was developed for use with extreme axial length cases to maximize the accuracy of predictions. For "average" eyes, constituting more than 75% of the total, the unmodified SRK formula may be used.

Stable postoperative refractive data were collected on 2,068 posterior chamber intraocular lenses (IOLs). The SRK II formula, although as simple as the unmodified formula, was comparable to, and in some cases better than, current second-generation formulas. Less than 1 D of prediction error was found for 80% of all lenses, and only 0.5% had 3 D or more of error. In short eyes, less than 22 mm, 74% were corrected to within 1 D. Of long eyes, 24.5 mm or more, 78% had less than 1 D of error. The mean absolute SRK II prediction error for the entire group was 0.64 D.

The SRK II is incorporated in most new A-scan units, but it is possible to take standard SRK predictions and mentally calculate modifications for extreme cases. The standard SRK formula suffices for eyes having axial lengths of 22.0 mm to 24.5 mm. The SRK II alters emmetropia predictions for only 1 of 4 patients with IOLs to be operated on.

▶ Intraocular lens power calculation with the original SRK formula is a safe alternative to compare against the "computer" and is easy to use. The SRK II is a refinement that should further improve the IOL power required to correct very small eyes and large eyes.—R.E. Adams, M.D.

---

**Long-Term Course of Surgically Induced Astigmatism**
Richards SC, Brodstein RS, Richards WL, Olson RJ, Combe PH, Crowell KE (Univ of Utah)
*J Cataract Refract Surg* 14:270–276, May 1988                    1–8

Corneal astigmatism may continue to change for years after intraocular surgery. Induced astigmatism was studied in 229 patients with extracapsular cataract extraction and posterior chamber lens implantation. The average follow-up was 2.9 years.

*Procedure.*—A 150-degree limbal groove 0.75 thick was made and a beveled 2-step incision created. After removing the nucleus and remaining cortex and implanting the lens, the limbal incision was closed with 10–0 nylon sutures. The intraocular pressure was adjusted to 15 mm Hg before a Terry keratometer was used to bring the corneal curvature to about 2.50 D of with-the-rule astigmatism. One to 3 sutures were cut in the axis of the plus cylinder in the first 4–7 weeks if there was more than 2.50 D of astigmatism.

Astigmatism increased to 1.65 D on initial postoperative study and then decreased gradually and was not significant after 2–3 years. The decrease was most rapid in the first months but continued for several years. Cutting sutures at 4–7 weeks did not influence the pattern of astigmatic change.

Few sex- or age-related differences were evident. In patients with no significant astigmatism shortly after surgery, against-the-rule astigmatism eventually developed when sutures were not cut. Patients with against-the-rule astigmatism after 3–4 years had less with-the-rule astigmatism in the early postoperative period.

These findings may not apply to operations involving short incisions or scleral tunnelling. Surgically induced astigmatism continued to change for at least 3 years. Consequent refractive shifts often are visually significant. Postoperative astigmatism does not return to its preoperative level. Long-term postoperative astigmatism depends chiefly on the type of incision made and the tightness of the sutures. Preoperative astigmatism has only a minimal effect on the final outcome.

▶ I tell my patients who are undergoing cataract surgery that glasses will be prescribed about 3 months after surgery. Surgically induced refractive changes decrease during the first 6 weeks. Scleral tunnel incisions and perioperative therapy with steroids help to decrease postoperative astigmatism, but ocular tissues particularly dislike surgical trauma, which causes swelling, stretching, and resultant astigmatism.—R.E. Adams, M.D.

---

### Relation of the Depth of the Anterior Chamber to the Lens Thickness: Clinical Significance

Olbert D (Univ Eye Hosp, Mainz, West Germany)
*Ophthalmic Res* 20:149–153, 1988                                   1–9

---

The relation of the depth of the anterior chamber to lens thickness and to the size of the globe was investigated, and a comparative analysis of the anterior eye segment was done, in 293 patients.

A relatively steady decrease in depth of the anterior chamber from 30 years on and a corresponding increase in lens thickness were noted. The average reduction in depth of the anterior chamber was 0.5 mm and increase of lens thickness 0.7 mm. An unexpected steadiness of the changes in the anterior eye chamber and of lens thickness, although in an inverse sense, was found. The distance between the anterior surface of the lens in women was, on average, 0.19 mm smaller than in men.

These findings confirm the known relationship between the depth of the anterior chamber and lens thickness. The age-related reduction in the anterior chamber was 1/3.5 on average.

▶ Annual axial length measurements of hyperopic eyes with shallow anterior chambers has been criticized as not cost effective and exploiting Medicare. Nevertheless, ultrasound is an objective basis for laser iridectomy, unlike slit-lamp biomicroscopy or gonioscopy.—R.E. Adams, M.D.

---

### Prophylactic Treatment of Intraocular Pressure Elevations After Neodymium:YAG Laser Posterior Capsulotomies and Extracapsular Cataract Extractions With Levobunolol

Silverstone DE, Novack GD, Kelley EP, Chen KS (Yale Univ; Univ of California, Irvine; Allergan, Inc, Irvine, Calif)
*Ophthalmology* 95:713–718, June 1988                                    1–10

Anterior segment surgery often is complicated by intraocular pressure elevation, even in patients with normal baseline pressure. A pressure rise after neodymium:yttrium/aluminum/garnet (Nd:YAG) capsulotomy may threaten vision. Various ocular hypertensive agents may help but often only transiently. Topical 0.5% levobunolol was evaluated in 2 double-masked, placebo-controlled studies of nonglaucomatous patients having lens-related surgery. Levobunolol is a $\beta_1$-, $\beta_2$-adrenoceptor antagonist and an effective ocular hypotensive agent.

Forty-two patients received levobunolol or vehicle 1 hour before unilateral Nd:YAG laser posterior capsulotomy. Thirty-eight percent of control patients and no treated patients had a pressure rise of at least 10 mm Hg. The mean intraocular pressure rose by up to 6 mm Hg in the vehicle recipients and decreased up to 3 mm Hg in treated patients. In the second study, 41 patients underwent unilateral extracapsular cataract extraction with a viscoelastic preparation and placement of a posterior chamber lens. Significant intraocular pressure rises occurred in 40% of control patients and in 19% of those given levobunolol.

Levobunolol may have a longer-lasting prophylactic effect than timolol in this setting. Although the drug minimizes intraocular pressure elevation, close monitoring of the pressure remains necessary.

▶ Elevated intraocular pressure after YAG capsulotomy is well documented. It is comforting to have another effective agent, levobunolol, to offset ocular pressure rise. Nevertheless, many will prefer Propine or Diamox because of potential systemic side effects with potent $\beta$ blockade.—R.E. Adams, M.D.

---

## Effect of Visual Blur on Contrast Sensitivity: Clinical Implications

Marmor MF, Gawande A (Stanford Univ Med Ctr)
*Ophthalmology* 95:139–143, January 1988                                    1–11

Little effort has been made to correlate the results of visual acuity and contrast sensitivity testing. Contrast sensitivity was measured under conditions of refractive blue producing specific acuity levels in 11 normal persons with corrected acuity of 20/20 or better. The age range was 16–64 years. Measurements were made at distances with Vistech charts, at near with Arden gratings, and with a pinhole to control pupil size.

When visual acuity was reduced by spherical lenses, contrast sensitivity declined over a broad range of spatial frequencies. These observations were made over all conditions. Even a modest refractive degradation of acuity in normal individuals results in a broad loss of contrast sensitivity.

It may be hazardous to interpret contrast sensitivity findings in patients with reduced acuity relative only to standard contrast sensitivity values if these are based on persons with normal visual acuity. If the possible effect of acuity is considered, contrast sensitivity testing can distinguish between deficits roughly equivalent to the acuity loss and those indicative of more distinct pathologic conditions.

▶ Reduction of contrast sensitivity occurs in ophthalmic disease, especially clouding of the ocular media. Rapid clinical evaluation of cataract is possible using an inexpensive and simple test system consisting of low-contrast letters.— R.E. Adams, M.D.

## Glare Disability as a Cause of Deterioration of Vision in Cataract Patients

Sjöstrand J, Abrahamsson M, Hård AL (Sahlgren's Hosp, Göteborg, Sweden)
*Acta Ophthalmol (Copenh)* 65:103–106, 1987                                    1–12

Cataract patients often are troubled by glare conditions, making it important to evaluate glare disability preoperatively in patients with turbid ocular media. Because slit-lamp study gives information only on back-scattered light and standard acuity testing does not reflect daily conditions, glare disability was quantified by contrast sensitivity testing and the use of low-contrast letters (E F K N U V X Y). Patients with varying degrees of cataract in 1 or both eyes but no other ocular disease were studied. Testing was conducted under glare conditions.

The use of low-contrast letters to document glare deficits was faster and easier than previously used methods. Increased turbidity of the ocular media is related to more marked glare disability, but the latter correlates only weakly with visual acuity. The effect of intraocular transfer of glare disability from a cataractous eye is marginal. Glare disability assessment is important in the preoperative study of patients with turbid ocular media.

▶ The principle of refractive error correction to improve the visual acuity applies to contrast sensitivity testing. Modest refractive degradation of acuity in normal persons results in a broad loss of contrast sensitivity. This differs from interferometry and retinal visual potential.— R.E. Adams, M.D.

## Correlation Between Intraoperative and Early Postoperative Keratometry

Masket S (Canoga Park, Calif)
*J Cataract Refract Surg* 14:277–280, May 1988                                    1–13

The value of intraoperative keratometry in limiting postcataract astigmatism has not been proved. Accurate readings require control of certain variables, including intraocular pressure. Whether quantitative intraoperative keratometry correlates with early postoperative office measurements if intraocular pressure is kept constant at surgery was investigated. In patients having cataract extraction by phacoemulsification with posterior chamber lens implantation, final suture tension adjustment and keratometry were done either at uncontrolled pressure levels or with the intraocular pressure standardized at 15 mm Hg.

Uncontrolled patients had a mean 2.15 D of with-the-rule cylinder on quantitative keratometry at the end of surgery, compared to 2.06 D with the pressure controlled, an insignificant difference. The mean corneal cylinder, measured by office keratometry the next day, was similar in both groups. The difference between intraoperative and postoperative keratometry was significant only in the uncontrolled group. Mean intraocular pressure 1 day after surgery was similar in the 2 groups.

Careful control of surgical variables, notably intraocular pressure, reveals positive correlation between intraoperative keratometry and 1-day postoperative office measurements. The greater the surgically induced with-the-rule cylinder, the greater the astigmatic decay after operation. It is best to limit the iatrogenic intraoperative cylinder to provide for early, stable, visual recovery from cataract surgery. Intraoperative keratometry can promote this goal by avoiding iatrogenic swings in corneal astigmatism.

▶ Intraoperative keratometry increases surgical time but can ensure against tight or loose sutures. Experience helps. Conventional "corneal" wound closure requires extreme care in suture placement and tension. This is opposed to scleral pocket or tunnel wound, which has helped me avoid "iatrogenic astigmatism."—R.E. Adams, M.D.

---

**Clinical Endothelial Cell Loss Following Phacoemulsification and Silicone or Polymethylmethacrylate Lens Implantation**
Levy JH, Pisacano AM (New York Eye Surgery Ctr, Bronx)
*J Cataract Refract Surg* 14:299–302, May 1988                    1–14

---

Endothelial cell loss reportedly is greater with phacoemulsification than with extracapsular or intracapsular cataract extraction. Significant cell losses are described with polymethylmethacrylate (PMMA) implants. The results of implanting 160 PMMA lenses were compared with those of 104 silicone lens implantations following phacoemulsification in the posterior chamber. Viscoelastic solution was used in all procedures. All silicone implants were of the ciliary sulcus type. Corneal endothelial cell counts were made 3–12 months postoperatively.

The mean reduction in endothelial cell count after PMMA implantation was 16.4%. Twelve percent of eyes had a decrease exceeding 1,200 cells/sq mm. The mean fall in cell counts after silicone implantation was 23.3%, and 15% of patients had a decrease of over 1,200 cells/sq mm. From 2% to 3% of patients in each group had an increase of more than 0.6 mm in central pachymetry. Cell losses after silicone lens placement were less on flat insertion than when a folding-bar inserter or a syringe-style inserter was used.

Endothelial cell loss is related more to the type of procedure than to the type of implant used. Proper surgical technique is critically important. Folding insertion methods must be improved if endothelial cell damage is to be reduced to levels seen with the flat insertion technique.

▶ Flexible soft intraocular lenses (IOLs) require special folding devices. Current instruments are awkward and unpredictably release the IOL, resulting in damage to the corneal endothelium. Improved insertion technique is essential, or the foldable IOL will be associated with postoperative "bad corneas."—R.E. Adams, M.D.

**Cataracts Induced by Microware and Ionizing Radiation**
Lipman RM, Tripathi BJ, Tripathi RC (Univ of Chicago)
*Surv Ophthalmol* 33:200–210, November–December 1988          1–15

There is increasing use of microware radiation, which is at the low-frequency end of the electromagnetic spectrum. Cataract induction by microwave radiation is apparent in rabbits and dogs, but human case reports are more controversial. Both anterior and posterior subcapsular opacities have been observed, with the former developing sooner after the start of exposure. Vacuolation of outer lens fibers and nuclear pyknosis have been described.

Both elevation of temperature and decreased levels of ascorbic acid in lenses have been related to microwave-induced lens changes. Elevation of temperature may be necessary but not sufficient to produce cataracts. Thermoelastic expansion may produce direct damage in the lens including formation of globules and holes in cell membranes.

X-ray-induced cataracts have been demonstrated in a variety of experiments. Worgul monitored the development of subcapsular opacities in the exposed frog eye, starting with the formation of large vacuoles in the posterior cortex and later in the anterior cortex. Formation of cataracts has been related to damage in the lens cell membrane or damage to the lens cell DNA, or both.

Different forms of radiation are able to induce formation of cataracts by distinct mechanisms that include damage to the cell membrane, formation of free radicals, and breaks in DNA bonds. Heat and ionizing radiation may complement each other in their effect on lens cells, as they do in destroying tumor cells.

**Observations on Lens Epithelial Cells and Their Removal in Anterior Capsule Specimens**
Hara T, Hara T (Hara Eye Hosp, Utsunomiya, Japan)
*Arch Ophthalmol* 106:1683–1687, December 1988          1–16

A wide part of the central anterior lens capsule is removed at cataract surgery. The cell density and the size of the lens epithelial cells were studied in 49 anterior capsules removed from patients who had routine phacoemulsification for cataract. A 7-mm round piece of central anterior capsule was removed and placed in a balanced salt solution. Twenty-five additional senile cataractous eyes were subjected to various procedures before removal of epithelial cells. These included simple aspiration, aspi-

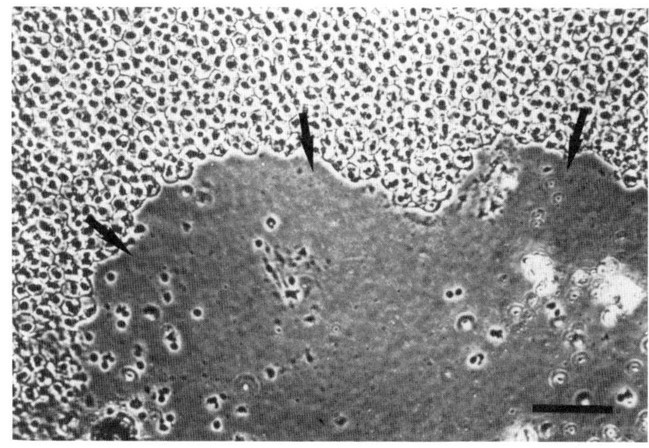

Fig 1–6.—Anterior capsule treated with single cryopexy application. Lens epithelial cells are thoroughly destroyed *(arrows)*. Cell debris is observable in treated area. *Bar* indicates 100 μm; ×40. (Courtesy of Hara T, Hara T: *Arch Ophthalmol* 106:1683–1687, December 1988.)

ration with ultrasound, single and double cryopexy applications, and double cryopexy followed by ultrasound aspiration.

The cell density of cataractous eyes declined with advancing age, and cell size increased with age. Simple aspiration removed cells almost completely, whereas aspiration with ultrasound completely removed the cells. A single cryopexy application could destroy the cell structure completely (Fig 1–6). The most effective treatment was double cryopexy followed by ultrasound aspiration; the cells were totally removed without debris remaining.

Long-term transparency can be achieved by either killing the cells or removing them completely. Cryopexy probably is a more secure method than ultrasound aspiration. The tip of the cryoprobe may be applied from the outer surface of the anterior capsule. It is best to remove debris by aspiration with ultrasound after application of cryopexy.

## Ocular Perforation From a Retrobulbar Injection

Schneider ME, Milstein DE, Oyakawa RT, Ober RR, Campo R (White Mem Med Ctr; Univ of Southern California, Los Angeles)
*Am J Ophthalmol* 106:35–40, July 1988                1–17

Data were reviewed on 7 patients who had ocular perforation from retrobulbar injection leading to acuity of 20/200 or worse. Proliferative vitreoretinopathy occurred in 3 patients. Two patients had direct macular injury and 2 had macular pucker. In all cases the needle injury exit site was in the posterior pole. Associated conditions included axial myopia, multiple injections, previous retinal buckling surgery, and enophthalmos.

Five perforations preceded cataract extraction. Sharp disposable 25-gauge or 27-gauge, 1¼-in. or 1½-in. needles were used in 6 patients, and a 23-gauge Atkinson nondisposable needle in 1. Five eyes were operated on. One patient had argon laser photocoagulation of the perforation site, and 1 patient was untreated. Final acuity was hand motions in 3 patients, largely because of recurrent detachment secondary to proliferative vitreoretinopathy. Two patients had a final acuity of 20/40 or better.

Serious complications of retrobulbar injection are being reported increasingly often. The superotemporal gaze position is dangerous. If retrobulbar anesthesia is required, a modified intraconal technique or an extratenons peribulbar injection may be relatively safe. All patients given retrobulbar anesthesia should have ophthalmoscopy within 10 days.

▶ Careful retrobulbar injection has proved through the years to be an effective and safe procedure. The patient should not look upward but, rather, keep the eyes in a straight-ahead gaze to avoid posterior perforation. The effectiveness of peribulbar injection compared to retrobulbar injection has not been proved; most surgeons prefer to stay with the traditional retrobulbar injection for efficacy and safety.

A careful parallel comparison study to assess the advantages and disadvantages of each procedure certainly is called for.—P.R. Laibson, M.D.

---

**Drugs, Including Alcohol, That Act as Risk Factors for Cataract, and Possible Protection Against Cataract by Aspirin-Like Analgesics and Cyclopenthiazide**
Harding JJ, van Heyningen R (Univ of Oxford, England)
*Br J Ophthalmol* 72:809–814, November 1988                                      1–18

---

A case-control study of cataract enrolled 300 cases and 609 controls aged 50–79 years to identify factors associated with cataract formation. An increased risk of cataract was associated with steroids (including the diuretic spironolactone), nifedipine, heavy cigarette smoking, and heavy beer drinking. The use of aspirin-like analgesics such as ibuprofen, paracetamol, and aspirin itself appeared to protect against cataract. Cyclopenthiazide also had an apparent protective effect.

Aspirin-like drugs were used for a variety of reasons by these patients. A protective effect of the drugs themselves is more likely than an effect of the disease for which they are taken. Acetylation of lens proteins possibly protects these proteins against chemical insults such as cyanate, glucose, and prednisolone that are associated with cataract. Alternatively, aspirin-like analgesics lower blood glucose levels.

Prevention of cataract may be an additional reason for the use of low-dose aspirin or paracetamol. Many persons already use these drugs to prevent myocardial infarction and stroke.

# 2  Cornea

## The Cornea and External Disease

Elisabeth J. Cohen, M.D.
*Cornea Department, Wills Eye Hospital, Philadelphia, Pennsylvania*

In cornea and external disease certain subjects are always important, such as herpes simplex keratitis, others that are issues of current concern (e.g., *Acanthamoeba* keratitis), and many diseases that fall in between.

In the area of herpes the major current issues concern the role of systemic antivirals and topical corticosteroids in treatment. Systemic acyclovir ameliorates the acute course of herpes zoster keratitis, although it does not appear to affect postherpetic neuralgia (1). High-dose systemic acyclovir has rapidly become accepted as part of the standard treatment of acute herpes zoster ophthalmicus.

Herpes simplex virus is also sensitive to acyclovir. Studies have documented the efficacy of topical acyclovir in the treatment of dendritic herpetic keratitis (2). However, it was not found to be superior to vidarabine. Acyclovir is not available as an ophthalmic topical medication in the United States. Systemic acyclovir has been used to prevent recurrent herpes simplex infection in immunocompromised patients and to treat primary ocular herpes simplex infection in adults.

The value of systemic acyclovir in recurrent herpes simplex keratouveitis has been the subject of uncontrolled studies (3). With the approval of the Herpetic Eye Disease Study (HEDS), the value of systemic acyclovir in recurrent herpetic keratouveitis will be studied in a well-designed, randomized, controlled, multicenter clinical trial.

In this study, the role of topical corticosteroids in the management of herpetic keratouveitis will also be investigated. The subject of corticosteroids in herpes simplex keratitis has been characterized by controversy with significant regional differences of opinion. There has been agreement that topical corticosteroids aggravate an episode of acute dendritic keratitis and are contraindicated in this stage of herpes. However, strongly held opposing views exist regarding topical corticosteroids for stromal keratouveitis. One opinion is that the adverse effects of topical corticosteroids for stromal keratitis outweigh potential benefits. The other opinion is that judicious use of topical corticosteroids can reduce the inflammation and scarring associated with stromal keratitis even though improper use can be complicated by progressive corneal melting and perforation. It is a major undertaking to try to clarify this issue through a multicenter randomized clinical trial.

The HEDS study applies valid epidemiologic and statistical methods to assess different treatments of herpes simplex keratitis, a common cause of unilateral blindness secondary to corneal disease in the United States today. Randomized clinical trials are expensive, time-consuming endeavors, but are necessary to obtain valid data regarding optimal treatment of common, important diseases. Randomized clinical trials regarding treatment of diabetic retinopathy have provided fundamental information concerning the indications for laser treatment. Randomized clinical trials are powerful research tools that are difficult to design, get funded, and complete. Ophthalmologists should try to aid in the recruitment of appropriate patients for the HEDS study and other randomized clinical trials in ophthalmology.

During the 1980s, microbial keratitis associated with soft contact lens use has been an important subject. Early correct diagnosis and treatment are important in the management of corneal ulcers (4). The clinical impression is that the risk associated with extended-wear soft contact lenses is greater than the risk associated with daily wear soft contact lenses. This question is difficult to answer because of problems determining the number of people wearing extended and daily wear lenses at risk. During 1988, research was conducted to try to determine the relative risk of extended versus daily wear. In one study, FDA data contained in premarket approval applications was retrospectively reviewed to determine the relative risk of sight-threatening adverse reactions. In another investigation sponsored by the Contact Lens Institute, a prospective case control study was conducted to address this same issue. The results of both studies have not yet been published by early 1989. Information regarding preliminary data analysis suggests that both studies will document increased risk associated with extended wear lenses.

The introduction of disposable lenses has been accompanied by optimism that this modality may reduce the complications associated with extended-wear cosmetic soft contact lenses (5). Disposable lenses are to be worn for 1 week and then discarded. Problems caused by infrequent disinfection prior to reinsertion of lenses, contaminated lens solutions, and old coated lenses should be reduced with disposable lenses. However, these lenses are the same as previously approved extended-wear lenses repackaged for disposable usage and are associated with hypoxia when the eyes are closed during sleep. Another question regarding these lenses is whether or not they will be used correctly according to the manufacturer's recommendation by the lens-wearing general public. Reports of complications associated with disposable lenses are beginning to appear in the literature. It will be interesting to see how these and similar lenses meet the test of time and customary usage as compared to the experience reported during short-term investigations.

*Acanthamoeba* keratitis remains an important problem even though it is uncommon because both medical and surgical treatment have limited efficacy. Various early manifestations have been reported recently including dendritiform keratitis (6) and epithelial lines (7) in addition to radial keratouveitis (8). It is important to suspect and diagnose this potentially disastrous infection before the typical ring infiltrate develops. Early diagnosis and treatment may improve the prognosis. Promising results using clotrimazole in combination therapy for both primary and recurrent infections were published in 1988 (9). This is encouraging news. Other investigators, however, have observed that clotrimazole was not effective against *Acanthamoeba* cysts (10). Due to the great problems in the therapy of *Acanthamoeba* keratitis, prevention remains of paramount importance.

In an excellent paper, significant risk factors for *Acanthamoeba* keratitis among contact lens wearers were determined to include use of homemade saline, infrequent disinfection, and swimming with contact lenses (11). Education is necessary to improve the compliance of contact lens wearers with recommended lens care regimens including regular disinfection prior to insertion. In addition to improper lens care, use of contaminated solutions has been linked with microbial keratitis among lens wearers (12). Legally, lens solutions are required to be sterile when open. Unfortunately, with regard to homemade saline, the device regulated by the FDA is the salt tablet and not the solution, made from nonsterile distilled water, which is actually used for lens care. Contrary to the recommendations of the Ophthalmic Device Panel of the FDA, the American Academy of Ophthalmology, and the Contact Lens Institute, the FDA has put forth educational material regarding correct use of homemade saline in a Safety Alert at the end of 1988. However, homemade saline will not be used as suggested only before and during heat disinfection because lens wearers frequently rinse their lenses with saline after disinfection prior to insertion.

The saline used for lens care must at least be sterile when opened and use of fresh commercial saline is recommended to further reduce solution contamination. Salt tablets should not be available for use with contact lenses. It is important for ophthalmologists to educate their lens patients not to use salt tablets or distilled water in caring for lenses and to disinfect lenses regularly prior to insertion.

*References*

1. Cobo LM, Foulks GN, Liesegang T, et al: Oral acyclovir in the therapy of acute herpes zoster ophthalmicus. *Ophthalmology* 93:763–770, 1986.
2. Laibson PR, Pavan-Langston D, Yeakley WR, et al: Acyclovir and vidarabine for the treatment of herpes simplex keratitis. *Am J Med* July 20, 281–185, 1982.
3. Schwab IR: Oral acyclovir in the management of herpes simplex ocular infections. *Ophthalmology* 95:423–430, 1988.
4. Stein RM, Clinch TE, Cohen EJ, et al: Infected vs. sterile corneal infiltrates in contact lens wearers. *Am J Ophthalmol* 105:632–636, 1988.
5. Donshik P, Weinstock FJ, Wechsler S, et al: Disposable hydrogel contact lenses for extended wear. *CLAO* 14:191, 1988.
6. Lindquist TD, Sher MA, Doughman DJ: Clinical signs and medical therapy of early acanthamoeba keratitis. *Arch Ophthalmol* 106:73–77, 1988.
7. Florakis GJ, Folberg R, Krachmer JH, et al: Elevated corneal epithelial lines in acanthamoeba keratitis. *Arch Ophthalmol* 106:1202, 1988.
8. Moore MB, McCalley JP, Kaufman HE, et al: Radial keratoneuritis as a

presenting sign in *Acanthamoeba* keratitis. *Ophthalmology* 93:1310, 1986.

9. Driebe WT Jr, Stern GA, Epstein RJ, et al: Acanthamoeba keratitis: Potential role for clotrimazole in combination chemotherapy. *Arch Ophthalmol* 106:1196–1201, 1988.

10. Osato MS, Robinson NM, Wilhelmus KR, et al: Cysticidal activity of 21 antimicrobial agents against 11 corneal isolates of *Acanthamoeba*. *Invest Ophthalmol Vis Sci* 29(suppl):40, 1988.

11. Stehr-Green JK, Bradley TM, Brandt FH, et al: *Acanthamoeba* keratitis in soft contact lens wearers. *JAMA* 258:57, 1987.

12. Bowden FW, Cohen EJ, Arentsen JJ, et al: Patterns of lens care practices and lens product contamination in contact lens associated microbial keratitis. *CLAO* 15:49, 1989.

---

## Oral Acyclovir in the Management of Herpes Simplex Ocular Infections

Schwab IR (West Virginia Univ, Morgantown)
*Ophthalmology* 95:423–430, April 1988                    2–1

---

Herpes simplex keratitis still is the most frequent cause of corneal blindness in developed countries, and little progress has been made in treating deep stromal and uveal involvement. The oral antiviral agent acyclovir was evaluated in 27 patients with ocular herpes simplex virus (HSV) infection. Twenty patients were treated acutely for active stromal keratitis, with or without uveitis. Four patients were treated after intraocular surgery, and 4 received the drug as coverage during withdrawal of other treatment. Twenty-one patients had multiple recurrences previously. The dose of acyclovir was 200 mg 5 times daily for 2 or 3 weeks, followed by tapering to 2 or 3 times daily.

All patients with active stromal keratitis or keratouveitis responded to acyclovir therapy, but 1 relapsed on tapering of treatment. Active epithelial defects nearly always resolved within 3 weeks. There has been only 1 recurrence during 194 cumulative months of treatment, and this followed a dose reduction. Twenty-four of all 27 patients improved, remained free of disease, or successfully had topical therapy tapered while taking acyclovir.

Oral acyclovir is a promising approach to HSV stromal keratitis and keratouveitis, particularly in immunosuppressed patients. Its prophylactic use has been effective in operated-on patients. Acyclovir probably limits HSV replication postoperatively, and this may be important when prolonged steroid therapy is necessary after corneal transplantation. Deeper disease such as herpetic keratouveitis continues to be difficult to treat.

▶ Oral acyclovir may prove to be helpful in the management of refractory herpes simplex keratouveitis. Further studies evaluating this treatment are necessary.—E.J. Cohen, M.D.

**Infected vs. Sterile Corneal Infiltrates in Contact Lens Wearers**
Stein RM, Clinch TE, Cohen EJ, Genvert GI, Arentsen JJ, Laibson PR (Wills Eye Hosp, Philadelphia)
*Am J Ophthalmol* 105:632–636, June 1988                                   2–2

Clinical impressions are relied on when deciding whether to obtain corneal scrapings or to initiate antimicrobial therapy in contact lens wearers having corneal infiltrates. Fifty patients with untreated infiltrates were studied prospectively in an attempt to distinguish clinically between infected and sterile infiltrates. If infection was suspected, patients were treated with topical fortified tobramycin and cefazolin. Otherwise, regular-strength tobramycin was used.

Initially, 30 patients were though to have infected infiltrates, and 20 patients, sterile corneal infiltrates. Pain and photophobia were the most prevalent initial symptoms. Seventeen of 20 culture-positive patients had moderate to severe discomfort. Discharge was seen only in infected eyes, but 3 eyes with small bacterial ulcers lacked discharge. The size of the infiltrate was less predictive of its nature. All culture-positive patients and only 7 of 20 patients with negative cultures had an epithelial defect. Moderate or severe anterior chamber reaction characterized culture-positive cases. Half of the culture-positive cases were associated with *Pseudomonas*. Two patients with *Pseudomonas* ulcers and 1 with *Acanthamoeba* keratitis lost more than 2 lines of visual acuity.

Corneal infiltrates associated with significant pain, anterior chamber reaction, discharge, and an overlying epithelial defect should be scraped for smear and culture, and managed as if infected. If a sterile infiltrate is likely, discontinuance of lens use and regular-strength topical antibiotics will suffice. Patching is contraindicated.

▶ Corneal ulceration is the most serious complication associated with soft contact lenses. *Pseudomonas* ulcers are most common among persons wearing cosmetic soft lenses. This article analyzes the presenting symptoms and signs associated with infected compared to sterile infiltrates. The clinician evaluating a patient with a history of contact lens use and a corneal infiltrate should suspect infection, perform cultures, and begin fortified antibiotics if significant pain, anterior chamber reaction, discharge, or an overlying epithelial defect is present.—E.J. Cohen, M.D.

---

***Acanthamoeba* Keratitis: Potential Role for Topical Clotrimazole in Combination Chemotherapy**
Driebe WT Jr, Stern GA, Epstein RJ, Visvesvara GS, Adi M, Komadina T (Univ of Florida, Gainesville; Rush-Presbyterian-St. Luke's Med Ctr, Chicago; Div of Parasitic Diseases, Centers for Disease Control, Atlanta)
*Arch Ophthalmol* 106:1196–1201, September 1988                          2–3

Clotrimazole, an antifungal agent, has excellent in vitro activity against most strains of *Acanthamoeba*. It was used in treatment of 4 patients

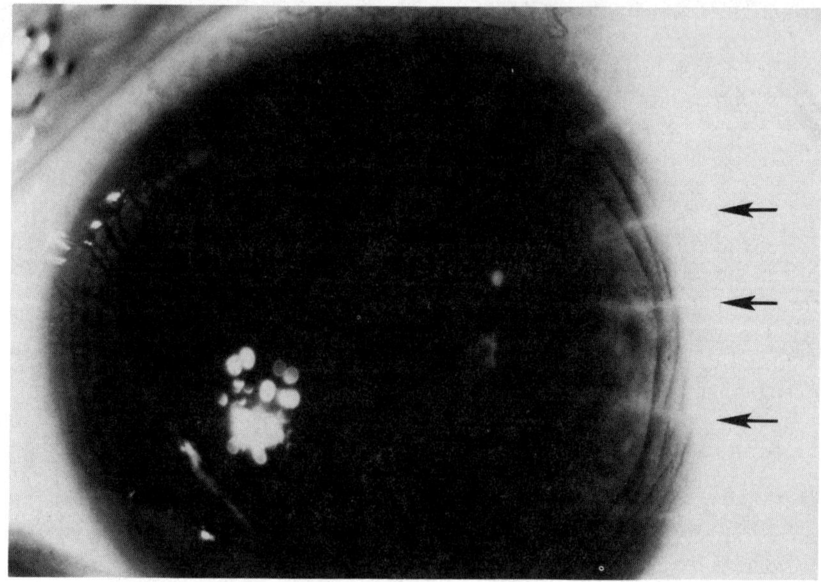

**Fig 2–1.**—Radial keratoneuritis *(arrows)* was noted at initial presentation. (Courtesy of Driebe WT Jr, Stern GA, Epstein RJ, et al: *Arch Ophthalmol* 106:1196–1201, September 1988.)

who contracted *Acanthamoeba* keratitis while wearing contact lenses stored in homemade saline solution (Fig 2–1).

Medical treatment regimens included the use of topical 1% clotrimazole. In 2 patients in whom conventional therapy failed, clotrimazole was successful in controlling recurrent infection after penetrating keratoplasty. Two other patients were given clotrimazole plus propamidine isethionate and neomycin sulfate–polymyxin B sulfate–gramicidin from the beginning and had an excellent response to treatment. Patients who found the commercially available cream uncomfortable were able to tolerate a 1% clotrimazole suspension formulated in artificial tears.

*Acanthamoeba* keratitis was successfully treated with topical 1% clotrimazole in 4 patients. The results demonstrate that topical 1% clotrimazole can be helpful in controlling this disease in some cases.

▶ *Acanthamoeba* keratitis remains a most difficult diagnostic and management problem. It can result not only in loss of vision but also in loss of the eye and prolonged morbidity. Topical clotrimazole can be effective in refractory primary and recurrent *Acanthamoeba* infections. This drug has relatively low minimal inhibiting concentrations and minimal amebicidal concentrations. Prevention of *Acanthamoeba* keratitis through use of commercially prepared contact lens solutions, proper contact lens disinfection, and avoidance of swimming with contact lenses in place remains critical.—E.J. Cohen, M.D.

**Clinical Signs and Medical Therapy of Early *Acanthamoeba* Keratitis**
Lindquist TD, Sher NA, Doughman DJ (Univ of Washington; Univ of Minnesota)
*Arch Ophthalmol* 106:73–77, January 1988                    2–4

Three patients had a dendritiform epithelial pattern early in the course of *Acanthamoeba* keratitis, which probably represents epithelial infection before any stromal involvement. Early diagnosis with wide epithelial débridement and medical treatment eradicated the protozoan. Keratoplasty was necessary in 1 of 2 other patients in whom the infection was not diagnosed until significant stromal involvement was present.

When the diagnosis was made within several weeks of onset of symptoms, a dendritiform epithelial pattern was observed. This may explain why many patients are treated for herpes simplex keratitis before the correct diagnosis is made. However, frank stromal keratitis was not present. The involved epithelium has an edematous and necrotic appearance. There may be mottled epithelial staining or frank defects, but often the epithelium appears intact. Once a fully developed ring-shaped infiltrate is present, there generally is extensive stromal involvement by amebic keratitis.

Broad epithelial débridement can debulk the infectious and immunogenic load of *Acanthamoeba*. Topical propamidine isethionate, Neosporin, and miconazole nitrate in addition to débridement are effective when the infection is diagnosed early. One of the patients in whom the diagnosis was made late successfully underwent penetrating keratoplasty; in another, a corneal perforation developed.

▶ Dendritiform keratitis is an early manifestation of *Acanthamoeba* keratitis. Recognition of early *Acanthamoeba* keratitis is very important to increase the chances of successful medical therapy of this potentially devastating infection.—E.J. Cohen, M.D.

---

**Selection of Controls for Clinical Research Studies in Ophthalmology**
Hawkins BS (The Johns Hopkins Med Inst, Baltimore)
*Arch Ophthalmol* 106:835–840, June 1988                    2–5

If controls are taken from the same ophthalmology clinic or practice as the cases in a trial, the groups will be similar, but the controls may not be representative of the general population. The problem arises in retrospective case-control studies and in prospective cohort studies. When cases and controls are matched, the factors used in matching cannot be investigated in the study. Community controls most often are obtained through random digit dialing, but this can produce a group of persons who are home during the usual workday.

A case-control study done in Washington County, Maryland, in 1970 and a later 15-year cohort study of the same subjects provided an opportunity to examine controls obtained from different sources. Participation rates were higher for office patients selected for study in both the case-control and cohort studies. In the cohort study, office controls were more likely to lose visual acuity and have degenerative eye disorders. Seven new cases of age-related macular degeneration and 2 cases of other degenerative diseases were diagnosed in office controls, but none were diagnosed in population controls.

Although more office patients may participate in research studies, they may not be representative. The use of more than 1 control group lowers the chance that differences between cases and controls are a result of referral patterns or of the need for evaluation or treatment. An investigator, when in doubt, may study control groups selected from more than 1 source to be sure that important biases have not been overlooked. Consultation with a biostatistician or epidemiologist during the design phase of a study is helpful.

▶ The importance of statistics and epidemiology in the planning and conducting of valid clinical research cannot be overemphasized. The use of controls is necessary in most well-designed studies, and the selection of appropriate controls is discussed in this paper. Consultation with a biostatistician during the early planning stages of a clinical research project is very helpful. The annual Epistat course presented by the National Eye Institute provides an excellent introduction to the role of epidemiology and biostatistics in clinical research.— E.J. Cohen, M.D.

**Controlling Risks of the Possible Transmission of Human Immunodeficiency Virus**
Notice of American Academy of Ophthalmology: Clinical Alert
*Ophthalmology* 96:1–9, January 1989                                    2–6

Protective measures for all parties were considered by a committee established jointly by the American Academy of Ophthalmology, National Society to Prevent Blindness, and Contact Lens Association of Ophthalmologists. Protection of patients involves hand washing and adequate disinfection of instruments. Gowns and masks are not required for the usual ophthalmic examination. Tonometers may be cleaned with an alcohol sponge, but the use of bleach reduces or eliminates all human immunodeficiency virus (HIV) infectious agents. Instruments are cleaned with alcohol if used for a patient with infectious disease. Contact lenses must be disinfected between patients.

Hand washing between eye examinations is an important general precaution against infection in the office. Disposable gloves should be available for all health care workers, but gloves do not substitute for hand washing. Protective eyewear is not needed unless splashing with blood or blood-contaminated fluid is anticipated.

No-touch techniques of tissue handling minimize direct contact with tissues. Instruction in the proper handling of needles can prevent needle stick injuries. During surgery, needles are handled only with needle-holders.

The risk of contracting HIV infection in ophthalmic health care is remote. There is no evidence that the virus is acquired from tears. Adherence to these guidelines, however, will protect against other more infectious agents that may be present in patients with acquired immunodeficiency syndrome. In addition, nonphysician health care workers who have minimal knowledge of infection control will be protected. Like all physicians, ophthalmologists are obligated to provide care to all patients.

## The Identification and Incidence of Human Immunodeficiency Virus Antibodies and Hepatitis B Virus Antigens in Corneal Donors

Conway MD, Insler MS (Tulane Univ; Lousiana State Univ)
*Ophthalmology* 95:1463–1467, October 1988                    2–7

The question of whether human immunodeficiency virus (HIV) can be transmitted by transplantation of corneas from HIV-infected donors has become a serious concern. Two screening techniques have been used to detect corneal donors infected with HIV—a profile of high-risk persons and HIV seropositivity demonstrated by enzyme-linked immunosorbent assay. The findings of such screenings were studied to determine the incidence and demographic profiles of seropositive donors.

Forty eye banks responded to a questionnaire about screening of patients at risk for acquired immunodeficiency syndrome (AIDS) and hepatitis B. Respondents accounted for 26% of the total volume of eye donors in 1986 in North America. Of 8,787 donors, 60 (0.68%) had HIV antibodies, and 69 (1.33%) of 5,187 donors tested positive for hepatitis B virus. Age, cause of death, and source of tissue were also considered. The finding of seropositivity for HIV in very young and elderly donors without identified risk factors emphasizes the need to screen all potential cornea donors for the presence of HIV antibodies.

Of the HIV-seropositive donors, 46% were older than 50 years of age and presumably had no symptoms. This is an age group generally not considered at high risk for AIDS. Donors aged 1–20 years, another group considered not at high risk, accounted for another 9% of HIV-seropositive donors. Thus about 73% of the HIV-seropositive donors had no known risk factor.

▶ Seropositivity for HIV was rare (0.68%) among corneal donors in this series. Screening of all donors is necessary, however, because positive results were obtained in both young and elderly donors without known risk factors. Concern regarding the HIV status of corneal donors is appropriate. However, there have not been any cases reported to date of transmission of HIV by corneal transplantation. Hepatitis B seropositivity was found in 1.38% of potential donors.— E.J. Cohen, M.D.

## The Treatment of Postoperative Endophthalmitis: Results of Differing Approaches to Treatment

Stern GA, Engel HM, Driebe WT Jr (Univ of Florida, Gainesville)
*Ophthalmology* 96:62–67, January 1989

2–8

The treatment of endophthalmitis has improved markedly, but appropriate treatment of individual patients often is uncertain. Twenty-six patients with early or late postoperative endophthalmitis were treated in 1983 through 1986. All patients had at least 1 intravitreal injection of antibiotic. Gentamicin and either cefazolin or vancomycin were used initially. Steroids were used systemically in 18 cases and intravitreally in 7. Five patients had immediate vitrectomy and 7 had delayed vitrectomy.

The most frequent operation preceding endophthalmitis was extracapsular cataract extraction with posterior chamber lens placement (Table 1). Bacteria were isolated in 19 instances (Table 2). Twenty patients were cured of infection. Five had recurrent infections, and 1 eye failed to respond to treatment. Two of the eyes that were cured became phthisical, and 1 patient required enucleation because of chronic irritation. Eleven of 12 patients who had vitrectomy were cured, but in 2 of these patients phthisis developed. All culture-negative patients were cured by a single intravitreal injection of antibiotics. Eight of the 10 patients with infection caused by *Staphylococcus epidermidis* were cured. Only 2 of 8 patients infected by virulent organisms recovered useful vision, but some of these patients had poor preexisting acuity.

Culture-positive patients with endophthalmitis may require repeated intravitreal antibiotic injections or vitrectomy, or both. Any episode of endophthalmitis has the potential to be devastating. Vitrectomy is considered as part of the initial management in severely affected eyes, those with levels of hypopyon greater than 15%, or those in which vitreous

TABLE 1.—Surgical Procedures
Preceding Endophthalmitis*

| Surgical Procedure | No. of Patients Treated |
|---|---|
| ECCE with PC IOL implantation | 15 |
| ICCE with AC IOL implantation | 3 |
| ICCE | 1 |
| Filtering surgery for glaucoma | 3 |
| Secondary IOL implantation | 1 |
| Discussion of pupillary membrane | 1 |
| Penetrating keratoplasty | 1 |
| Strabismus surgery | 1 |

*ECCE, extracapsular cataract extraction; PC, posterior chamber; IOL, intraocular lens; ICCE, intracapsular cataract extraction; AC, anterior chamber.

(Courtesy of Stern GA, Engel HM, Driebe WT Jr: *Ophthalmology* 96:62–67, January 1989.)

TABLE 2.—Bacteria Identified as Cause of Endophthalmitis

| Organism | Early Post-operative Period | Late Post-operative Period | Total |
|---|---|---|---|
| *Staphylococcus epidermidis* | 9 | 1 | 10 |
| *Staphylococcus aureus* | 0 | 1 | 1 |
| *Streptococcus pneumoniae* | 0 | 1 | 1 |
| Alpha-hemolytic streptococcus | 1 | 1 | 2 |
| Group D streptococcus | 1 | 1 | 2 |
| *Propionibacterium acnes* | 0 | 1 | 1 |
| *Pseudomonas aeruginosa* | 1 | 0 | 1 |
| *Proteus mirabilis* | 1 | 0 | 1 |
| Culture-negative | 5 | 2 | 7 |

(Courtesy of Stern GA, Engel HM, Driebe WT Jr: *Ophthalmology* 96:62—67, January 1989.)

opacification obscures the red reflex. Eyes affected mildly or moderately, and have negative cultures, may do well after initial intravitreal antibiotic injection.

## The Effect of Suture Removal on Postkeratoplasty Astigmatism

Binder PS (Sharp Cabrillo Hosp, San Diego)
*Am J Ophthalmol* 105:637—645, June 1988                                  2–9

Follow-up was made of 439 eyes for at least 6 months after corneal transplantation with placement of 8 interrupted 10–0 sutures and a single, continuous 16-bite 11–0 nylon suture. All sutures were removed from 188 eyes on an average of 20 months after operation. Central keratometry readings and keratographs were used to determine which interrupted sutures to remove. Sutures were removed from an eye with less than 3 D of astigmatism only when hyperopia was present and corneal steepening was required. Suture removal began 6 weeks postoperatively.

A single wound leak occurred after removal of an interrupted suture, and it sealed spontaneously. Thirty-five eyes required contact lenses to achieve best corrected acuity. The mean corneal astigmatism was 3.7 D before suture removal and 3.5 D afterward, not a significant change. About one fourth of eyes had 1 D or more of increased astigmatism following suture removal. Astigmatism decreased more in eyes with greater than 5 D of presuture removal astigmatism. Astigmatism was not a function of donor-recipient disparity.

Selective suture removal can reduce astigmatism after corneal transplantation while sutures are in place. Rapid recovery of visual acuity is possible, compared with the removal of all sutures before a final spectacle prescription. In addition, astigmatism is reduced. When sutures are left in place for 18 months or longer, a more stable wound results and there is less change in corneal curvature when the sutures are removed.

▶ The use of a combined interrupted and running suture technique for penetrating keratoplasty has been a significant advance. In addition to enabling early selective suture removal to reduce astigmatism, there are other advantages compared to the use of a running suture. It is easier to keep the chamber deep during the procedure, the running suture does not need to be tightened as much, and wound closure is stronger.—E.J. Cohen, M.D.

## Effect of Donor Epithelium on Corneal Transplant Survival

Stulting RD, Waring GO III, Bridges WZ, Cavanagh HD (Emory Univ)
*Ophthalmology* 95:803–812, June 1988                                    2–10

Because epithelial cells express large amounts of class I histocompatibility and Langerhans' cells express class II antigen, removal of donor epithelium at the time of penetrating keratoplasty might promote graft survival through limiting rejection. This hypothesis was examined in a series of 232 penetrating keratoplasties in 228 eyes. Randomly selected patients had their grafts rubbed with cellulose sponge until no epithelium remained. Topical antibiotics and steroids were used routinely. Allograft reactions were treated with topical forms of steroids and, in some cases, oral forms.

Graft survival after more than 2 years postoperatively was 91% when the epithelium was left on and 81% when it was removed. The respective rates of irreversible rejection were 2.7% and 4.1%. Allograft reactions did not differ significantly in frequency in the 2 groups. Removal of the epithelium did not delay the onset of allograft reactions.

Previous studies of the effect of removing donor epithelium have given conflicting results. Patients at high risk of rejection were excluded from the present study, which showed a higher overall failure rate when the epithelium was removed. The removal of donor epithelium does not enhance graft survival in penetrating keratoplasty or lower the risk of rejection.

▶ This is a well-designed clinical study providing evidence that removal of the corneal epithelium does not reduce the risk of rejection. If the epithelium is in good condition, it would appear best to leave it in place.—E.J. Cohen, M.D.

## Accuracy and Precision of the Tono-Pen in Measuring Intraocular Pressure After Keratoplasty and Epikeratophakia and in Scarred Corneas

Rootman DS, Insler MS, Thompson HW, Parelman J, Poland D, Unterman SR (Louisiana State Univ)
*Arch Ophthalmol* 106:1697–1700, December 1988                            2–11

The Goldmann and Schiotz tonometers do not give reliable readings of intraocular pressure when the cornea is irregular, and the MacKay-Marg tonometer no longer is in production. The Tono-Pen is a hand-held tonometer that operates on the same principle as the MacKay-Marg instrument. Multiple pressure measurements are made, and average and confidence levels are displayed in a readout.

Both the MacKay-Marg and Tono-Pen tonometers were used to record intraocular pressure in 37 eyes with irregular corneas, which were most often caused by corneal edema or scarring, and in 50 eyes that recently had undergone penetrating keratoplasty. Sixteen eyes that had undergone epikeratophakia and 12 with normal corneas also were examined. Five investigators collected the data.

Analysis of variance showed no significant difference between measurements made with the 2 instruments in any group. If a pressure of greater than 21 mm Hg obtained with the MacKay-Marg instrument was taken as abnormal, the Tono-Pen produced 3 of 46 false positive results for a sensitivity of 93% and 6 of 69 false negative results for a specificity of 91%.

The Tono-Pen is essentially as accurate as the MacKay-Marg tonometer in measuring pressure in eyes with scarred and irregular corneas. It is those eyes in which pressure measurement is most difficult that require the closest monitoring. The Tono-Pen is convenient to use and the disposable latex tips used with the device ensure sterility. This instrument may actually work in a greater range of ocular disorders than the MacKay-Marg tonometer.

---

**Effect of Long-Term Contact Lens Wear on Corneal Endothelial Cell Morphology and Function**
Carlson KH, Bourne WM, Brubaker RF (Mayo Clinic and Found, Rochester, Minn)
*Invest Ophthalmol Vis Sci* 29:185–193, February 1988          2–12

---

A number of studies have shown significant endothelial changes in long-term contact lens wearers. Age-related changes in the corneal endothelium and its limited regenerative potential make these findings of concern. Studies were made in 40 patients aged 17–42 years who had worn contact lenses for at least 2 years and in 40 controls of similar age. All study subjects had a negative ophthalmologic history and normal ocular findings.

There was no marked difference in endothelial permeability or central corneal thickness beween the lens wearers and controls. The mean cell size was reduced in the lens wearers, and the coefficient of variation of cell size was increased in this group. None of the morphological or functional variables could be related to years of lens wear or duration of daily lens wear.

Contact lens wear does affect the corneal endothelium. If corneal hypoxia is responsible, a lens providing adequate oxygen to the cornea should be best, but this remains to be confirmed. The endothelial cell changes appear to develop early and to regress slowly. There is greater variation in endothelial cell size and shape than in controls but no differences in endothelial function are apparent.

▶ Studies in endothelial morphology to detect variations in cell size (polymegathism) and cell shape (pleomorphism) are helpful in detecting evidence of endothelial instability. In long-term contact lens wearers, changes occur in endothelial morphology.—E.J. Cohen, M.D.

## Corneal Endothelial Changes Associated With Herpetic Stromal Keratitis

Hirose N, Shimomura Y, Matsuda M, Inoue Y, Inaba M, Hamano T, Manabe R (Osaka Univ Med School, Japan)
*Jpn J Ophthalmol* 32:14–20, 1988                                      2–13

Focal disorder of the corneal endothelium is associated with the stromal lesions of herpetic keratitis. Computerized specular microscopy was used to detect subtle endothelial changes in 33 patients having unilateral herpetic stromal keratitis, none of whom had a history of other ocular disease. Sixteen patients had disuiform keratitis alone and 17 had at least 1 episode of keratouveitis.

In patients with disuiform keratitis only, increased variation in cell size and shape was apparent in the affected eye. These changes were more marked in patients with keratouveitis, and endothelial cell density was reduced in these patients. In both groups the proportion of hexagonal cells was reduced in affected eyes compared with fellow eyes.

Substantial changes are found in the corneal endothelium in patients with herpetic disuiform keratitis and keratouveitis. Polymegathism and pleomorphism are characteristic findings. Endothelial cell density is lowered in eyes affected by keratouveitis. There may be ongoing stress or damage to the corneal endothelium after herpetic keratitis. Both viral invasion of endothelial cells and an attack of immunocompetent cells against the endothelium are possible pathogenetic mechanisms.

▶ Endothelial morphology studies suggest that abnormalities are present in patients with resolved disuiform keratitis. Patients with herpes keratouveitis have evidence of greater endothelial insult and cell loss. This technique is being used to evaluate the endothelium in a wide variety of diseases.—E.J. Cohen, M.D.

## Topical Retinoid Therapy for Squamous Metaplasia of Various Ocular Surface Disorders: A Multicenter, Placebo-Controlled Double-Masked Study

Soong HK, Martin NF, Wagoner MD, Alfonso E, Mandelbaum SH, Laibson PR, Smith RE, Udell I (Univ of Michigan; Washington Hosp Ctr, Washington, DC; Massachusetts Eye and Ear Infirmary, Boston; Univ of Miami; Manhattan Eye and Ear Infirmary; et al)
*Ophthalmology* 95:1442–1446, October 1988                             2–14

Preliminary studies of tretinoin showed clinical improvement in symptoms and visual acuity, rose bengal staining, and Schirmer test results in patients with keratoconjunctivitis sicca (KCS) and ocular cicatricial diseases. There was also histologic evidence that squamous metaplasia was reversed by the drug. This preliminary study, however, was not double masked and placebo controlled and the number of subjects was limited. Thus a randomized, double-masked, multicenter, placebo-controlled study was done to assess the efficacy and safety of tretinoin in the treatment of dry eyes in 161 patients. Of these, 116 were observed for a minimum of 4–8 months, qualifying them for final statistical analysis.

Analysis of adjusted mean changes in KCS showed no significant differences between the active treatment and placebo groups. A similar analysis of patients with conjunctival cicatricial diseases showed a significant reversal of conjunctival keratinization in the temporal bulbar site after treatment with active drug. However, clinical symptoms and signs showed no significant improvement with active drug compared with placebo. Side effects, limited to blepharoconjunctivitis, were reversible on tapering or cessation of the drug.

Topical ophthalmic tretinoin is not effective in improving the signs and symptoms of noncicatricial dry eyes. However, the drug may have some therapeutic promise in reversing ocular surface keratinization in cicatricial diseases of the ocular surface.

▶ Topical tretinoin, a vitamin A analogue was not effective in the treatment of keratoconjunctivitis sicca in a placebo-controlled, double-masked study. Such studies are necessary to determine efficacy. Investigator bias may have been a factor in previous favorable open-label reports regarding this therapy.—E.J. Cohen, M.D.

---

## Use of Collagen Corneal Shields in the Treatment of Bacterial Keratitis

Sawusch MR, O'Brien TP, Dick JD, Gottsch JD (Wilmer Ophthalmological Inst, Johns Hopkins Hosp)
*Am J Ophthalmol* 106:279–281, September 1988                2–15

---

The collagen corneal shield, originally developed as a corneal bandage after radial keratotomy, keratorefractive procedures, and corneal abrasions, is fabricated from porcine scleral tissue, which has a collagen composition closely resembling that of the human cornea. An animal model of *Pseudomonas* keratitis was used to compare treatment with topical tobramycin with and without the presence of a commercially available collagen corneal shield.

Pilot studies showed a significant 30-fold increase in penetration of tobramycin into the anterior chamber when a collagen shield was used. Twenty albino rabbit eyes were inoculated with *Pseudomonas aeruginosa* to produce stromal keratitis, and topical tobramycin dosing was done for 12 hours. Eyes with a collagen corneal shield in place were found to have a significant decrease in colony-forming unit counts, compared with treated eyes without a shield and with untreated control eyes.

The collagen corneal shield may have a role in enhancing antibiotic therapy of microbial keratitis. The shield may either increase delivery of topical antibiotics, providing high initial drug levels, or decrease the necessary dosing frequency.

▶ Collagen shields may prove to be an effective drug delivery system. Although animal studies are necessary, there always are problems in extrapolating from animal models. In addition, in this study, regular-strength tobramycin (3 mg/ml) instead of the standard fortified tobramycin (15 mg/ml) was used with and without collagen shields to treat *Pseudomonas* keratitis.—E.J. Cohen, M.D.

---

## Evaluation of Topical Cromolyn Sodium in the Treatment of Vernal Keratoconjunctivitis

Foster CS, The Cromolyn Sodium Collaborative Study Group (Massachusetts Eye and Ear Infirmary, Boston)
*Ophthalmology* 95:194–201, February 1988                                    2–16

Vernal keratoconjunctivitis (VKC) is a chronic or recurrent form of ocular allergy. Cromolyn sodium, a mast cell stabilizing agent, was evaluated in a double-blind, multicenter, placebo-controlled trial in 72 patients with a diagnosis of active bilateral VKC. A 4% cromolyn sodium ophthalmic solution was instilled—2 drops per eye, 4 times daily.

Eighteen of 65 evaluable patients required other ocular medication, and treatment was considered a failure; 7 had been actively treated with cromolyn sodium. Cromolyn treatment was significantly superior to placebo with respect to conjunctival injection, limbal edema, tearing, and symptom scores. Few side effects occurred, and, with a single exception, they did not require interruption of treatment. When only patients with a history of atopic disease were considered, cromolyn again gave superior results. Physician global assessments indicated that substantial control was achieved in 79% of cromolyn-treated patients and in 38% of the placebo-treated group, a significant difference.

These findings confirm the efficacy and safety of cromolyn sodium, used topically, in the treatment of VKC, especially in patients with a clear atopic history. The risks of long-term cromolyn therapy appear to be minimal. The prophylactic use of cromolyn sodium can provide nearly total relief of symptoms throughout the year in most patients with VKC.

▶ Cromolyn sodium has been shown in a controlled study to be safe and effective in VKC. Cromolyn is an important drug in the management of VKC because it has reduced the need for topical corticosteroid treatment.—E.J. Cohen, M.D.

### Immunodiagnosis of Adult Chlamydial Conjunctivitis

Sheppard JD, Kowalski RP, Meyer MP, Amortegui AJ, Slifkin M (Univ of Pittsburgh; Allegheny Gen Hosp, Pittsburgh)
*Ophthalmology* 95:434–443, April 1988                    2–17

Four available diagnostic tests for ocular *Chlamydia trachomatis* infection were compared in 76 patients suspected of having chlamydial conjunctivitis. Giemsa stain cytology, direct monoclonal fluorescent antibody (DFA) microscopy, and the enzyme immunosorbent assay (EIA) for chlamydial antigens were compared with the standard McCoy cell culture.

Twenty-two patients had at least 1 positive diagnostic chlamydial test result. Fifteen had a false positive EIA or DFA test result; they were younger than patients with negative test results and had been symptomatic for a shorter time. Enzyme immunosorbent assay testing correlated best with McCoy cell culture. The Giemsa, EIA, and DFA tests did not correlate closely with one another. Giemsa cytology had an overall accuracy of 67%. It effectively screened 67% of the study group, compared with 79% for the DFA test and 95% for both EIA and the Giemsa stain tests.

Immunodiagnostic methods do not depend on live organisms but, rather, rely on highly specific labeled antibodies to chlamydial surface antigens. The EIA correlated best with McCoy cell culture in the present study. The DFA test predicted the largest number of positive responses to antibiotic therapy. The Giemsa stain is rapid and specific but has limited sensitivity and requires skilled interpretation. The newer immunodiagnostic tests show considerable promise in diagnosing adult inclusion conjunctivitis. Dawson points out that topical antibiotic therapy interferes with the laboratory diagnosis of chlamydial conjunctivitis even if there is no substantial clinical response.

▶ New immunologic methods to diagnose *Chlamydia* infections are compared with the use of cell cultures and Giemsa stains. These new techniques are helpful because they are more readily available than cultures, but there is considerable variability in the results depending on the technique used.—E.J. Cohen, M.D.

---

### Treatment of Scleritis With Combined Oral Prednisone and Indomethacin Therapy

Mondino BJ, Phinney RB (Univ of California, Los Angeles)
*Am J Ophthalmol* 106:473–479, October 1988                    2–18

The initial recommended treatment for diffuse or nodular scleritis includes oral nonsteroidal anti-inflammatory drugs (NSAIDs). If a patient does not respond to these drugs, oral corticosteroids (e.g., prednisone) are recommended. Six patients with diffuse or nodular scleritis did not respond to oral doses of indomethacin or prednisone used alone but did respond when the drugs were used in combination.

The total daily doses of prednisone when used alone ranged from 40 to 100 mg; the total daily doses of indomethacin when used alone ranged from 100 to 200 mg. The use of combination therapy with prednisone in total daily doses of 10–60 mg and indomethacin in total daily doses of 50–150 mg resulted in a complete clinical response in these previously unresponsive patients. The corticosteroid-saving effect of NSAIDs permitted the use of lower doses of corticosteroids, thereby decreasing the risk of serious systemic side effects.

Combination therapy with NSAIDs and corticosteroids may be useful in patients resistant to either type of drug used alone.

▶ Standard treatment of scleritis has been the use of systemic NSAIDs *or* corticosteroids. This report suggests a new approach: combination therapy for scleritis, with improved efficacy despite reduced dosages of both drugs.—E.J. Cohen, M.D.

---

## Postoperative Instillation of Low-Dose Mitomycin C in the Treatment of Primary Pterygium

Hayasaka S, Noda S, Yamamoto Y, Setogawa T (Shimane Med Univ, Izumo, Japan)
*Am J Ophthalmol* 106:715–718, December 1988                    2–19

The efficacy of using 0.02% mitomycin C twice daily for 5 days after surgery was assessed in 80 patients who had primary pterygium treated in 99 eyes. Thirty-one eyes had excision of pterygium under topical anesthesia, leaving 3 mm of bare sclera adjacent to the corneoscleral limbus. Twenty other eyes had excision and postoperative β-radiation of the bare sclera. Nineteen eyes were treated with 0.04% mitomycin C 3 times daily for 1 week after operation, and 29 were treated with 0.02% solution twice daily for 5 days.

Thirty-two percent of eyes had recurrences after surgery only, as did 15% of irradiated eyes. The rate of recurrence was 11% with the use of the stronger mitomycin C solution and 7% with the weaker solution. Five of 19 eyes treated with the stronger solution had complications, including scleral ulceration without bacterial infection in 2. There was mild discomfort in 1 of 29 eyes when 0.02% mitomycin was used.

Postoperative instillation of 0.02% mitomycin C in saline appears to prevent recurrences of pterygium with infrequent complications. Systemic toxic effects have not occurred with this treatment.

---

## Successful Treatment of Postherpetic Neuralgia With Capsaicin

Bucci FA Jr, Gabriels CF, Krohel GB (Albany Med College, NY)
*Am J Ophthalmol* 106:758–759, December 1988                    2–20

Postherpetic neuralgia, a common complication of herpes zoster oph-thalmicus, is especially frequent in older patients. Current treatment methods have not been very successful, and the persistent, severe pain has led to marked depression and even suicide. The use of 0.025% capsaicin in the form of Zostrix topical analgesic cream was evaluated in 2 patients with a long history of postherpetic neuralgia who failed to respond to other treatment. Capsaicin presumably inhibits nociceptive impulses from the peripheral to the central nervous system.

A woman aged 72 years who had not responded to carbamazepine and amitriptyline gained nearly total relief of debilitating pain within 1 week when Zostrix was applied to the forehead and upper eyelid 4 times a day. A woman aged 65 years who had had postherpetic neuralgia for 7 months despite narcotic analgesics also had relief of pain within 1 week when Zostrix was applied. Both patients have continued to have relief from pain by using Zostrix.

---

## Citrate or Ascorbate/Citrate Treatment of Established Corneal Ulcers in the Alkali-Injured Rabbit Eye

Pfister RR, Haddox JL, Lank KM (AMI/Brookwood Med Ctr, Birmingham, Ala)
*Invest Ophthalmol Vis Sci* 29:1110–1115, July 1988                    2–21

---

The scorbutic state of new corneal fibroblasts following alkali injury to the eye might be reversed by exogenous ascorbate. Topical citrate also protects the rabbit cornea from ulceration and perforation when used immediately after alkali injury, presumably by inhibiting polymorph activity. The value of these measures in treating established corneal ul-cers was studied. Alkali injury was induced with 1 N NaOH in the rabbit eye.

Treatment with 10% citrate every 30 minutes significantly reduced the extent of anterior stromal ulcers. With combined 10% ascorbate and 10% citrate, there was only a trend toward a reduction in ulcer size. Only citrate-treated eyes showed significant improvement in heal-ing when compared with control eyes. Citrate alone also was most effective in preventing descemetocele or perforation. Treatment of poste-rior stromal ulcers did not prevent perforations in either treatment group.

Citrate treatment significantly improves healing in this rabbit model of alkali burn of the eye. Ascorbate is clearly less helpful in established cor-neal ulcers, possibly because few fibroblasts are present in the ulcer bed whereas citrate-inhibitable polymorphs are numerous. Citrate probably would be helpful in the clinical setting, because in vitro studies have dem-onstrated inhibition of human polymorphs.

▶ The treatment of severe alkali burns has always been difficult and frustrating for the ophthalmologist because of relentless corneal scarring, vascularization, and poor visual results. Even after the eye has quieted, corneal transplantation has a very poor prognosis in this disease. This article suggests that 10% citrate applied every half hour for 14 hours might be effective in ameliorating the severe collagen degradation and resultant scarring and vascularization. These authors have for years been attempting to find a way to manage severe alkali burns, and it appears that protection provided by citrate against deepening of established anterior corneal ulcers in alkaline-burned rabbits may be clinically meaningful and important.—P.R. Laibson, M.D.

## Vitamin A Eyedrops for Superior Limbic Keratoconjunctivitis

Ohashi Y, Watanabe H, Kinoshita S, Hosotani H, Umemoto M, Manabe R (Kansa; Rosai Hosp, Amagasaki, Japan; Osaka Univ)
*Am J Ophthalmol* 105:523–527, May 1988     2–22

Superior limbic keratoconjunctivitis is an intractable chronic inflammation seen chiefly in middle-aged women; it is of uncertain cause. Various treatments have been of inconsistent effectiveness in patients with this disorder. Twelve patients with superior limbic keratoconjunctivitis were treated with topical vitamin A eyedrops in the form of retinol palmitate. Ten patients (83%) responded after follow-up for 3 months or longer. Keratoconjunctivitis did not recur as long as topical applications continued.

The efficacy of topical vitamin A therapy in this study, although not as good as that of pressure patching and a soft contact lens, was nearly comparable to thermocauterization or conjunctival resection. Two patients who had failed to respond to silver nitrate had a good response to topical vitamin A therapy. Once remission occurred, the disease remained absent as long as treatment continued.

Vitamin A may be locally deficient in patients with superior limbic keratoconjunctivitis. It also is possible that topically applied vitamin A stimulates glycoprotein synthesis by the epithelium, with consequent modulation of the keratinization process. Topical vitamin A should be considered before surgery is undertaken for superior limbic keratoconjunctivitis.

▶ Ophthalmologists have desperately sought a treatment for superior limbic keratoconjunctivitis for many years. Although the authors report some success with vitamin A eyedrops, a better test would be a double-masked study using vitamin A eyedrops against a placebo. Because the symptoms and signs of superior limbic keratoconjunctivitis are so variable with remissions and exacerbations, only a well-designed study would really prove the efficacy of any single treatment as reported here. I would not rush out to treat my superior limbic keratoconjunctivitis patients with vitamin A drops based on these data.—P.R. Laibson, M.D.

## Topical Aminocaproic Acid Significantly Reduces the Incidence of Secondary Hemorrhage in Traumatic Hyphema in the Rabbit Model

Allingham RR, Crouch ER Jr, Williams PB, Catlin JC, Loewy DM, Jacobson J
(Eastern Virginia Med School, Norfolk)
*Arch Ophthalmol* 106:1436–1438, October 1988                    2–23

Secondary hemorrhage is a significant complication of traumatic hyphema. Because aminocaproic acid, an antifibrinolytic agent, lessens the risk of secondary bleeding when given orally, its topical use was evaluated in a rabbit model of traumatic hyphema. Hyphema was treated with a placebo gel of 4% carboxypolymethylene or with active gel, in a double-blind study, and both groups were compared with untreated control animals.

Both the placebo and control groups had a rebleeding rate of 33%, compared with only 10% in treated animals. The gel appeared to be well tolerated locally, and there was no evidence of systemic toxicity.

Topical aminocaproic acid may be an effective local measure for lowering the risk of secondary bleeding following traumatic hyphema. The visual prognosis should improve as a result. The gel preparation produces adequate concentrations of drug in the aqueous, and plasma levels are far lower than with systemic administration. Further toxicity studies are needed before clinical trials can be instituted.

▶ The use of aminocaproic acid topically rather than orally in secondary hemorrhage after traumatic hyphema may reduce the side effects of this treatment. This preliminary study in the rabbit model should be pursued further in humans if toxicity studies yield satisfactory results. The use of oral aminocaproic acid or other antifibrinolytic agents to reduce the incidence of secondary hemorrhage after traumatic hyphema is recommended until a better and safer drug is available. Also see Abstract 8–6 concerning the management of traumatic hyphema.—P.R. Laibson, M.D.

---

**Ocular Herpes Simplex Infection: Pathogenesis and Current Therapy**
Liesegang TJ (Mayo Clinic Jacksonville, Jacksonville, Fla)
*Mayo Clin Proc* 63:1092–1105, November 1988                    2–24

The expression of ocular herpes simplex disease depends on the site and extent of infection, host immunologic events, trophic damage within the ocular tissues, and the toxic effects of antiviral medications. Antiviral treatment is effective against some but not all aspects of the infection.

Acyclovir is the first relatively selective agent; it is phosphorylated by viral-induced thymidine kinase, an enzyme restricted to virus-infected cells. Acyclovir penetrates well into the aqueous and tears after intravenous or oral administration. Side effects of oral acyclovir are minimal. Nearly 30 clinical trials have confirmed the efficacy of topically administered acyclovir. Oral treatment may control deep or intraocular forms of infection.

Cycloplegics are used for herpetic infection of the corneal stroma. De-

---

Principles of Corticosteroid Use in Ocular Herpes Simplex Virus

- Avoid use of corticosteroids in active epithelial disease, trophic ulcers, and mild stromal keratitis
- Do not initiate topical corticosteroid therapy concurrently with initial antiviral treatment
- For stromal keratitis (necrotizing, diskiform, or interstitial) and uveitis, determine dosage of corticosteroid on the basis of severity of inflammation and interval since epithelial disease
- Avoid abrupt termination of corticosteroids; taper dose slowly by reduction in frequency or progressive dilution
- Use high-dose topical corticosteroid therapy after intraocular surgical procedures
- Maintain antiviral "cover" for corticosteroid use in excess of one drop of 1% prednisolone acetate/day. No antiviral "cover" needed with one drop of ⅛% prednisolone acetate/day

(Courtesy of Liesegang TJ: *Mayo Clin Proc* 63:1092–1105, November 1988.)

---

finitive conclusions on the efficacy of steroids are not yet available, but most types of disease do respond favorably (table). Steroid use should be avoided or tapered if there is dendritic or geographic keratitis, epithelial and stromal ulceration without stromal inflammation, or mild diskiform keratitis and iridocyclitis. In some cases tarsorrhaphy or a conjunctival flap may be indicated. If ocular perforation is imminent, cyanoacrylate glue and a contact lens or patch graft may salvage the globe for a later corneal transplant procedure.

# 3 Glaucoma

## Glaucoma Care—1988

Richard P. Wilson, M.D.
*Glaucoma Service, Wills Eye Hospital, Philadelphia, Pennsylvania*

I would like to discuss a potpourri of important aspects of glaucoma care that came into focus during 1988. As part of the total picture, Paul Palmberg has estimated the importance of glaucoma care in the national health picture. By his estimates, 80,000 Americans are blind from glaucoma. Two million persons in this country have the disease, although only half of them are aware of it. Five to 10 million people have increased intraocular pressure. Caring for known glaucoma patients requires 3.25 million office visits each year, about 8% of all the visits to the ophthalmologist.

New epidemiologic data is coming to light in the Baltimore Eye study. Al Sommer and The Johns Hopkins University have been conducting a thorough, well-designed glaucoma screening program in an urban setting with a higher proportion of black patients. In their study cohort, glaucomatous visual field defects were picked up in 3% of those screened, rather than the conventional 0.5%. The incidence of blacks with glaucoma compared with an age-matched group of whites revealed a 3- or 4-to-1 ratio. While the higher incidence of glaucoma in blacks has been suspected for many years from such sources as blind registries in America and screening programs in Africa, the Baltimore Eye Study is the first rigorously designed study to confirm these presumptions in this country. It now seems clear that blacks do have a higher incidence of glaucoma and, on average, contract the disease earlier. Like systemic hypertension, the disease seems to be more virulent in this group, or at least, the medications and surgical procedures available for treatment do not work as well for them.

Moving from epidemiologic to etiologic considerations, glaucoma has classically been defined as a triad of elevated intraocular pressure, characteristic disc, and visual field changes. Clearly, that waste basket disease classification, low tension glaucoma, did not fit in this definition. It was, therefore, the consensus of the 1988 American Glaucoma Society meeting that intraocular pressure should not be considered part of the definition of glaucoma. It is much more accurate to consider it a risk factor for the disease. Patients with an intraocular pressure of 10 mm are at risk for glaucoma, although the risk is small. On the other hand, patients with an intraocular pressure of 40 mm are at 100% risk if they live long enough. Intraocular pressure, therefore, can be considered a continuously increasing risk factor from an intraocular pressure in the single digits to the top of the measurable range.

As an example, glaucoma is much more akin to heart disease than polio. As serum cholesterol levels decrease, so does the risk of myocardial infarction. However, patients with low serum cholesterol levels still have heart attacks. With polio, on the other hand, if you eradicate the virus, the disease disappears. Therefore, intraocular pressure is a risk factor for glaucoma, but just one of them.

Other factors besides race have recently gained attention. A Japanese study has shown that with age there is a gradual increase in intraocular pressure similar to that seen in this country. However, once individuals with systemic hypertension and obesity are omitted from the studied population, the intraocular pressure average remains flat with increasing age. It therefore appears that systemic hypertension may be a risk factor.

Migraines are seen in 25% of the population, but Richard Lewis has shown that they are present in 48% of those with low tension glaucoma. It would, therefore, seem that vasospastic disease is a risk factor for at least low tension glaucoma. Other, more theoretical risk factors include a weak, floppy lamina cribrosa or abnormally large pores in the lamina giving poor support to the nerve axons. This could allow damage to the axons at a lower intraocular pressure level.

In dealing with a disease that has so many variables, it is always alluring to try to fit them all together in one pathophysiologic mechanism. This is dangerous as there are very likely at least two and probably more pathophysiologic mechanisms for glaucoma damage, just as there are many different etiologies for elevated intraocular pressure. Color vision testing provides part of my basis for this belief. There are some glaucoma suspects who develop yellow/blue axis color vision loss well before definite glaucomatous visual field change. Yet there are other patients with only a central island left who have normal color vision. Obviously, damage is occurring in different ways in these disparate groups.

The medical treatment of glaucoma has moved slowly ahead during the last year, but promises greater breakthroughs in the near future. In running through the different classifications of medical therapy, I would like to start with miotics. The pilocarpine Ocusert has been around for many years. There is little advertising for it, and many practicing ophthalmologists have lost sight of this little-used but very effective medication vehicle. Until thymoxamine becomes available, it is still the best treatment for young myopes with pigmentary glaucoma. The lesser amount of induced myopic shift compared with drop (pulsed) regimens is constant and can be corrected with a change in glasses.

Many physicians have been put off by the time-consuming job of explaining the product and its use to the patient. Alza has tried to counter this with instructional booklets and a video tape that can be used in the office. These explain to the patient how to use the Ocusert, its insertion and removal. Samples with and without pilocarpine are also available from Alza (800-277-9553, or in California call collect at 415-494-5067). Because the combination of a β blocker and miotic is our most potent topical combination, Ocuserts should be remembered when treating younger patients in whom a β blocker alone does not control the intraocular pressure.

In evaluating the β blockers, one has to consider effect, duration of effect, safety, and cost. Studies are fairly conclusive that timolol is equal to levobunolol and both are stronger than betaxolol. Roughly 10% of patients do not respond to β blockers at all. Although betaxolol usually will result in an intraocular pressure drop within 1 or 2 mm of that achieved by a nonselective β blocker, an additional 10% of those patients that respond to timolol or levobunolol will not respond to betaxolol.

Levobunolol lasts slightly longer than timolol, although both may be used once a day in glaucoma patients with easily controlled intraocular pressures. Betaxolol is strictly a twice-daily drug. If once-a-day usage is to be tried, the patients should be tested in the office 20 to 24 hours after the last installation to make sure the diurnal curve is being adequately controlled. The patient can then return to his every morning or every night dosage regimen.

The selective β blocker, betaxolol, is significantly safer than the nonselective blockers whether one is considering pulmonary, cardiac, central nervous system, or other systemic disease. The reasons for this are several, but chief among them is the specificity/affinity ratio of betaxolol. It is quite specific for $\beta_1$ adrenergic receptors (heart) but has much less affinity for those receptors than the nonselective β blockers. This means that a much higher concentration of betaxolol will be necessary to block even $\beta_1$ receptors compared with timolol although betaxolol is $\beta_1$ specific. The reason betaxolol is effective in the eye is the high intraocular concentration produced by 1 drop on the cornea.

I do not use betaxolol in asthmatic patients under medical treatment for their disease. I do, however, use it when other medical alternatives have been exhausted in patients with chronic obstructive pulmonary disease or a past history of asthma. Clearly, this needs to be done with the patient's awareness of possible complications and, when appropriate, the consent of their personal physician. Because asthma is an episodic disease, several trials of the medication to monitor symptoms, or the use of pulmonary function tests with and without the drug, are required to prove patient intolerance.

Levobunolol and betaxolol are similar in cost, and both are significantly less expensive in comparison with timolol. However, a group at UCLA has looked at the cost per dose, and their results are interesting. They found that a 10-ml bottle of timolol consistently contained 11.1 ml, while the same size bottle of levobunolol held only 10.1 ml. More importantly, the drop size of timolol, with its lesser viscosity and Ocumeter delivery system was 28 μL compared with 46 μL for the more viscous levobunolol. There were 1.77 times more drops per 10-ml bottle of timolol than levobunolol. Therefore, the authors figured that levobunolol would have to cost 56% less per equivalent bottle to be less expensive. The smaller drop size with timolol may affect the incidence of side effects and both considerations should be included in the physician's decision to prescribe a β blocker.

A word of caution needs to be injected here. For the above discussion to hold true, patients must use the Ocumeter dispensing system as intended. They must hold the bottle by the sides, but only press in on the bottom of the inverted bottle. If they squeeze the sides, the drop size will vary. In comparison, I have had several complaints from patients who, after inverting the levobunolol bottle, found the medication free-flowing into their eye, resulting in overdosage and waste.

My present approach (it changes with each new article read) when I intend to use a β blocker takes into account these considerations. If safety is a concern, I prescribe betaxolol. If I feel once-a-day usage is adequate and will enhance patient compliance, I employ levobunolol. If neither indication fits, I use timolol, preferably in the 0.25% concentration in whites, the 0.5% in blacks (see Abstract 3–11).

One mistake that I occasionally see in the resident clinic is the combination of dipivifrin (Propine) in combination with phospholine iodide or carbachol. Both are cholinesterase inhibitors, and dipivifrin requires an esterase to convert it to epinephrine, the active form. The above combination does not allow dipivifrin to be converted and it remains inactive.

Aplastic anemia, a rare but disastrous complication of carbonic anhydrase inhibitor use, has been brought to the fore by Frederick Fraunfelder. He has suggested, before therapy, screening with a complete blood cell (CBC) count patients who are to be given carbonic anhydrase inhibitors, and to do such screening every 6 months thereafter. Is this a reasonable directive to be employed on all patients? The consensus of the American Glaucoma Society is No! With slight simplification, there are two kinds of blood dyscrasias caused by carbonic anhydrase inhibitors. One is a dose-responsive bone marrow suppression. If treatment with the carbonic anhydrase inhibitors is stopped, the bone marrow recovers. Certainly, if this type of anemia is discovered early, the patient is less symptomatic, but complications are unusual. The other kind, aplastic anemia, is an idiosyncratic reaction and is 50% fatal no matter when it is discovered and how it is treated. Aplastic anemia can occur with the first dose (an important consideration for ophthalmologists who use Diamox routinely before or after cataract surgery) but usually during the first 2–3 months of treatment. It rarely occurs after 5 or 6 months. Discovering the dyscrasia with a CBC at an earlier time than would be possible with symptoms alone will not alter the final outcome. Therefore, far less impetus exists to obtain them. The problem is also exceedingly rare. It has been estimated that more patients would die in automobile accidents on the way to the lab for the blood test than would die of the disease itself. To my knowledge, routine CBCs to detect aplastic anemia are not done by any glaucoma specialist.

However, selected patients should have a CBC before the start of therapy. Because glaucoma patients are often elderly and sometimes infirm, there is an increased incidence of anemia in this population. It is disturbing to have a patient respond well to carbonic anhydrase inhibitors only to have to discontinue them when anemia is discovered later on a routine examination. If the anemia had been found and treated previously, carbonic anhydrase inhibitor treatment could be continued. Therefore, patients with a suggestive history or appearance would be well served by having a CBC before the start of treatment.

Topical carbonic anhydrase inhibitors have been under study for many years. At last, one of these has reached the testing stage. A 2% concentration of MK 927 lowers intraocular pressure significantly up to eight hours after application. Although this method of application would dramatically reduce the dose-responsive side effects inherent in carbonic anhydrase inhibitor use, it would not eliminate the idiosyncratic reaction, aplastic anemia. The ability, however, to use this medication in patients who are intolerant of oral carbonic anhydrase inhibitors would be of significant benefit.

The newest medication available for the treatment of glaucoma is apraclonidine (Iopidine). This is an $\alpha_{-2}$ agonist that decreases aqueous humor formation by approximately 35% without any effect on outflow. The main side effects have been nasal and oral dryness as well as conjunctival blanching. It has been approved to date for use in aborting the postoperative pressure rise often seen after laser trabeculoplasty and laser iridectomy. It remains to be seen whether this drug will be a helpful adjunct in long-term therapy or will suffer from tachyphylaxis, short-term escape, or long-term drift. One study by Morrison, however, has shown that when added to timolol apraclonidine produced an average 4.3-mm drop at 6 hours with a lesser but still significant additive effect at 22 days. This is a hopeful sign of possible future potential.

A more exciting possibility is the prostaglandin group. In uveitis, the uveoscleral outflow is increased by a factor of six, providing a drop in intraocular pressure as a backup for when the posterior trabecular meshwork is blocked by cellular debris. This increase in uveoscleral outflow is mediated by prostaglandins. When steroids are added, the prostaglandins are decreased and the uveoscleral outflow also decreases causing a rise in intraocular pressure. The increase in uveoscleral outflow appears to be secondary to the widening of spaces between the ciliary body muscle fibers and a decrease in intracellular substance. The isopropyl ester of prostaglandin $F_{2\alpha}$ is more lipophilic, and therefore a lesser dose is required. In a 0.001% solution, it causes a reduction in intraocular pressure that is evident by 4 hours and lasts up to 24 hours. There is no contralateral effect. The main side effect is conjunctival hyperemia, which can be extreme but variable. Burning, stinging, irritation and foreign body sensation are also possible.

The exciting aspect of this medication is that it does not work through decreasing aqueous production or increasing trabecular meshwork outflow. This agent is, therefore, not bound by episcleral venous pressure, which is usually around 9. In the monkey, in which approximately 50% of the outflow is through uveoscleral channels as opposed to the 10% to 20% in man, 1 drop of 0.001% prostaglandin $F_{2\alpha}$ can drop the pressure to 1 or 2. It is hoped that this medication would allow more effective treatment of low-tension glaucoma by lowering intraocular pressure into the very low ranges. Because it works by a mechanism totally different from any of our other medications except for atropine, and to a lesser degree epinephrine, it would be additive to the rest of our armamentarium.

On the surgical front, 1988 has seen growing support for the use of antifibrosing agents, silicone tube shunts, and cyclophotocoagulation of the ciliary body. The national multicenter trial investigating 5-fluouracil (5-FU) will conclude its investigation and release a report later this year. The report surely will be an anticlimax, because other investigators such as Robert Weinreb have shown its effectiveness, often with far lower doses and far fewer side effects than have been reported by the Miami group using the same protocol as in the national study.

The use of 5-FU postoperatively has certainly changed my practice. Many of the procedures that would have required a silicone shunt or a ciliodestructive procedure in the past can now be handled adequately with a trabeculectomy and 5-FU. Postoperative care is greatly expanded, however. I have found that the 48% epithelial erosion rate cited in the early Miami study can be dropped to approximately 20% if the certain recommendations are followed. No 5-FU is given at the close of procedure. This allows the cornea a day to recover from the drying effects of the operating room microscope. It also allows the surgeon to ensure that there are no leaks in the conjunctiva before the start of 5-FU therapy. I have been giving injections on day 1 and 2 postoperatively and 2 more within the first week. I give 3 injections in each of the next 2 weeks on a flexible schedule but spread out as much as possible. During the period when the 5-FU injections are given, I use ointments every 90 minutes during the day rather than topical drops. By keeping the cornea moist continuously, there is far less chance of corneal erosion. The hardship on the patient and his family, especially if they live a distance from the surgeon, is markedly increased by these frequent trips. However, the results justify this additional effort. Other antifibrosing agents such as aminoproprion-itrile are under investigation and may prove even more effective than 5-FU.

Silicone tube shunts employing either the Molteno implant or the Schocket shunt have gained wide acceptance. Neither of these devices has a pressure-sensitive valve implanted in the tube and therfore cannot be called valves. The effect is to shunt aqueous from the anterior chamber into the orbit by-passing the subconjunctival space. The shorter implants, such as the earlier Denver-Krupin valve, that ended in the subconjunctival space were subject to fibrosis of the conjunctiva to the sclera around the tube. This effectively eliminated the requisite area for aqueous absorption and caused frequent failure with these models. With the reservoir for the shunted aqueous placed posterior to the muscle insertions as is the case in the Molteno and Schocket procedures, this cannot happen. However, fibrosis around the reservoir can become thick enough to inhibit aqueous diffusion and result in failure. Still, the success rate with these shunts is in the 70% to 90% range, depending on which series you choose. This success rate is exceptional in these very recalcitrant eyes.

At present, for patients with inflammatory glaucoma, aphakic glaucoma in which there is no capsule to hold the vitreous back, neovascular glaucoma post PRP, and those with multiple failed filtering procedures, my approach is to use a trabeculectomy with releasable sutures converting the protected split-thickness procedure to a full-thickness procedure in the postoperative period. This procedure with postoperative injections of 5-FU is quite successful. If this combination fails, or if the patient comes from a great distance and the injections cannot be given by a local physician, a tube shunt is employed.

Physiologically, it seems much more appropriate to increase outflow rather than to destroy part of the eye to decrease inflow. A cyclophotocoagulation of the ciliary body ab externo with the continuous wave neodymium: yttrium/aluminium/garnet laser is my last choice. This procedure has also gained recognition in 1988. It is done either in a noncontact fashion with the Lasag unit, or with contact laser technology supplied by Surgical Laser Technologies. Both ways photocoagulate the ciliary body ab externo through the sclera and offer a 100% success rate at controlling intraocular pressure, although multiple procedures (one to four) may be necessary. The advantage of laser ablation of the ciliary processes compared with cyclocryotherapy is the smaller, more localized area of destruction with each application. This accounts for the much reduced pain and inflammation seen with laser cyclophotoablation. I have a 1% phthisis rate with up to 4 years' follow-up with this procedure, compared with 8% with cyclocryotherapy.

Although improved methods for treating glaucoma appear at an ever quicker pace, our understanding of the pathogenesis of the disease remains rudimentary. I hope that the coming year will shed more light on the etiology of glaucoma, the second leading cause of blindness overall and the leading cause of blindness in blacks.

---

**Early Trabeculectomy Versus Conventional Management in Primary Open Angle Glaucoma**
Jay JL, Murray SB (Univ of Glasgow)
*Br J Ophthalmol* 72:881–889, December 1988                    3–1

---

A prospective multicenter trial of conventional medical treatment and trabeculectomy enrolled 99 patients with previously undiagnosed primary open angle glaucoma. All had intraocular pressures of at least 26 mm Hg, along with field loss typical of glaucoma. The medical group received up to 3 different topical or systemic drugs. If pressure was uncontrolled or field loss progressed, trabeculectomy was carried out. Patients in the surgical group were operated on within a month of diagnosis.

Trabeculectomy was done in 53% of eyes in the medically treated group within 4 years. Surgery was done most often in patients with intraocular pressure above 30 mm Hg or substantial field loss with dense scotomas. Early surgery provided much more stable pressure control. The mean intraocular pressure after trabeculectomy was 15 mm Hg regardless of when surgery was done. Patients considered medically controlled had a mean pressure of 21 mm Hg after the first year. The visual fields were protected better by early surgery. Six patients in the medically treated group lost central fixation because of progressive field loss. Cataract developed in about 10% of the eyes, but it occurred earlier in medically treated patients.

Primary trabeculectomy appears indicated for patients with primary open angle glaucoma. An initial attempt at medical control merely delays surgery in many cases and the delay jeopardizes the visual fields. Surgery may be indicated especially when close supervision is not possible. Different considerations may apply to less advanced glaucoma.

---

**The Early Postoperative Pressure Course in Glaucoma Patients Following Cataract Surgery**
Vu MT, Shields MB (Duke Univ)
*Ophthalmic Surg* 19:467–470, July 1988                                        3–2

---

Patients with glaucomatous damage may be at risk of an early postoperative rise in intraocular pressure (IOP) after extracapsular cataract extraction (ECCE). The course of IOP in the first 2 months postoperatively was followed in 25 consecutive glaucomatous patients having extracapsular extraction, and in 25 others having intracapsular extraction without intraocular lens implantation. Patients having extracapsular extraction received a J-loop, angulated posterior chamber intraocular lens.

Half the patients undergoing ECCE had an IOP above 21 mm Hg on the first postoperative day. Eighty percent of this group had a pressure rise of at least 5 mm Hg, to levels above 21 mm Hg, within the first 26 days after surgery. The figure for patients having intracapsular extraction was 84%.

Savage et al. obtained similar findings. There is a slightly greater rate of early postoperative pressure rise after intracapsular extraction, but a significant number of eyes have a pressure rise after ECCE with posterior chamber lens implantation. All glaucoma patients should be closely followed after cataract extraction. If moderate or advanced glaucomatous damage is present, a conventional glaucoma procedure probably should be done before or in conjunction with cataract extraction.

▶ Many of the articles commenting on IOP after ECCE with posterior chamber lens implantation have correctly pointed out that the IOP 6 months to 1 year postoperatively is slightly less or the same as the preoperative IOP. One would conclude from this that it is safe to perform a standard ECCE in glaucoma patients if the IOP is controlled, whatever the glaucoma status. Vu and Shields point out that the early postoperative period is the most dangerous, especially as miotics and epinephrine compounds are usually contraindicated during this period. Therefore, patients who are already being treated with a β blocker and CAI may need a combined procedure or filtration surgery first, as the surgeon does not have a good way of dealing with a postoperative pressure spike, which could lead to further visual field loss.—R.P. Wilson, M.D.

**Treatment of Phacolytic Glaucoma With Extracapsular Cataract Extraction**
Lane SS, Kopietz LA, Lindquist TD, Leavenworth N (Univ of Minnesota; Univ of
Washington; Group Health Inc, St Paul)
*Ophthalmology* 95:749–753, June 1988                                      3–3

Intracapsular cataract extraction (ICCE) has classically been done to
treat phacolytic glaucoma. Extracapsular cataract extraction (ECCE) was
evaluated in 5 patients seen in 1984–1986. Extraction was followed by
placement of a posterior chamber intraocular lens. The surgery was uncomplicated and curative in all 5 patients. Intraocular pressures remained
below 20 mm Hg without medical treatment. All patients had a best corrected acuity of 20/50 or better on follow-up 5 months to 3 years after
operation.

Extracapsular cataract extraction with intraocular lens implantation is
an effective approach to phacolytic glaucoma. Care is needed to avoid
zonular rupture when performing the anterior capsulectomy. It is helpful
to flush proteinaceous material out of the eye and to instill a viscoelastic
material. All the patients reviewed were cured, and excellent acuity was
the rule. There is little evidence of serious complications from ECCE in
this setting. The present authors no longer consider ICCE as the preferred
operation for phacolytic glaucoma.

▶ Cataract extraction in the face of an inflamed eye with elevated IOP is always more difficult. Lane et al. show that an ECCE with a posterior chamber
intraocular lens is just as effective in relieving the secondary glaucoma as an
ICCE and offers a more satisfactory visual rehabilitation. Phacolytic glaucoma is
not the emergency that phacomorphic (secondary angle closure) glaucoma is.
Time should be taken to lower the intraocular pressure medically and quiet the
eye before intervention.—R.P. Wilson, M.D.

**Surgical Therapy of Chronic Glaucoma in Aphakia and Pseudophakia**
Gross RL, Feldman RM, Spaeth GL, Steinmann WC, Speigel D, Katz LJ, Wilson
RP, Varma R, Moster MR, Marks S (Wills Eye Hosp, Philadelphia)
*Ophthalmology* 95:1195–1201, September 1988                               3–4

Surgery is less effective in patients with uncontrolled aphakic or
pseudophakic glaucoma than in those with phakic glaucoma. A review
was made of the results of 91 initial glaucoma operations performed in
patients with aphakia from 1979 to 1986. Open-angle glaucoma was
present in 46 eyes and angle closure in 31. The most frequent procedures
were cyclodialysis, cyclocryotherapy, and argon laser trabeculoplasty. Patient mean age at operation was 63 years.

Successful surgery was defined as achieving an intraocular pressure of
less than 21 mm Hg and at least 30% lower than preoperatively, less
than 2 lines loss of acuity, and no need for further surgery. Using these
criteria, 4 of 15 patients had successful results from trabeculectomy after
9 months, and 3 of 20 from cyclodialysis. Only 1 of 8 patients responded

to cyclophotocoagulation with the neodymium: yttrium/aluminum/garnet (Nd:YAG) laser. Nine of 22 patients did well after cyclocryotherapy, and 2 of 20 after argon laser trabeculoplasty. Three of 6 patients responded to the Schocket procedure. Severe complications followed cyclocryotherapy and cyclodialysis.

These results are generally unfavorable and confirm the difficulty of surgery in aphakic glaucoma. No single procedure consistently lowers intraocular pressure and preserves vision. Only 25% of patients in this series had a successful outcome.

▶ This article confirms the poor success rate of glaucoma surgery in aphakic and pseudophakic patients. Although the study ended in 1986, it suggested that 1 silicone shunt procedure offered a better prognosis. In the intervening 2 years the use of the antimetabolite 5-fluorouracil as an adjunct to filtering surgery has proved effective in these difficult cases, and in the authors' practices is usually tried first. If not successful, it is followed by a shunt, and finally by cyclophotocoagulation of the ciliary body with the thermal mode Nd:YAG laser. These procedures have greatly increased the success rate and lowered the complication rate from those mentioned in the study.—R.P. Wilson, M.D.

---

**Medical Management of a High Bleb Phase After Trabeculectomies**
Scott DR, Quigley HA (Wilmer Ophthalmological Inst, Baltimore)
*Ophthalmology* 95:1169–1173, September 1988                         3–5

---

In some patients a high bleb and elevated intraocular pressure (IOP) develop after trabeculectomy. Both massage with topical steroids and surgery have been proposed. Eighteen such eyes were managed successfully with topical or systemic medications to decrease aqueous production. An encysted bleb developed in 10% of 181 eyes after simple trabeculectomy with a limbus-based conjunctival flap and tenonectomy. No blebs developed in 69 eyes after trabeculectomy with a fornix-based flap combined with extracapsular cataract extraction.

Long-term control of IOP was achieved in all 18 eyes. Medication was discontinued in 14 instances. Most of the eyes were treated initially with a topical β blocker. In several cases an oral carbonic anhydrase inhibitor also was used. Intraocular pressure usually became normal with 1–5 weeks.

In an eye disposed to the development of a high bleb, the IOP may rise when aqueous flow returns to normal after trabeculectomy. The bleb cavity expands but is limited laterally by healing at the surgical zone. Fluid movement through the bleb wall may not be adequate (Fig 3–1). Medical treatment reduces compression of the bleb wall, allowing the fluid channels to function fully. Pressure-lowering agents may not suffice in eyes with high IOP but no high bleb.

▶ The encapsulated bleb, Tenon's capsule cyst (a misnomer because there is no endothelial or epithelial lining), igloo syndrome, or whatever the name ap-

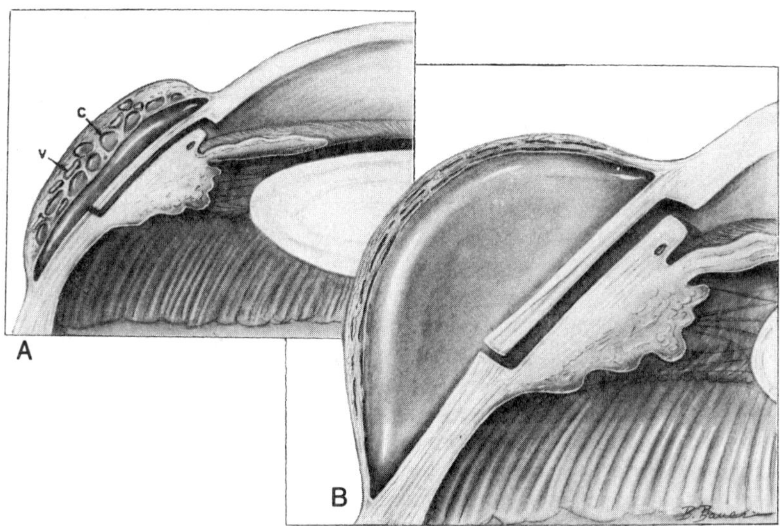


Fig 3–1.—**A,** normal trabeculectomy with microcystic spaces and vessels in the bleb wall. The blood vessels *(V)* and microcystic spaces *(C)* in the bleb wall are open, permitting movement of fluid out of the bleb. **B,** high bleb with compressed microcystic spaces and vessels in the bleb wall. The blood vessels and microcystic spaces have been compressed by the abrupt elevation of intraocular pressure. Movement of fluid out of the bleb is impaired. (Courtesy of Scott DR, Quigley HA: *Ophthalmology* 95:1169–1173, September 1988.)

plied, is best treated with medication rather than surgery so long as the IOP can be controlled well enough to prevent further optic nerve damage. In my experience, 2–4 months may be required for the encapsulation to resolve to the extent that aqueous is allowed to percolate through the wall and be absorbed. At that time, antiglaucoma medication should be reduced as much as IOP control will allow. Surgical intervention may result in the appearance of another encapsulated bleb and has not been necessary in this author's last 2,300 trabeculectomies.—R.P. Wilson, M.D.

## Transpupillary Argon Laser Cyclophotocoagulation in the Treatment of Glaucoma

Shields S, Stewart WC, Shields MB (Duke Univ)
*Ophthalmic Surg* 19:171–174, March 1988                    3–6

Transpupillary photocoagulation of ciliary processes using the argon laser has been proposed as an alternative to conventional glaucoma surgery. Adequate gonioscopic visualization permits the precise application of laser energy to individual ciliary processes without damaging adjacent structures.

Twenty-seven patients whose glaucoma was not controlled by maximal tolerated medication and standard laser methods underwent transpupillary argon laser cyclophotocoagulation. Only six (22%) had a successful outcome. Many patients had a further sustained rise in intraocular pressure (IOP) postoperatively. The average increase in IOP in 18 failures was 7.7 mm Hg. The elevation usually occurred within the first month after laser treatment. Two patients in whom treatment failed had decreased vision in the early postoperative period.

The success rate of transpupillary photocoagulation with the argon laser was low in this series. Apart from the number of ciliary processes visualized and treated, inadequate laser burns may be a factor in the outcome. The chief limitation may be the angle at which the ciliary processes are visualized gonioscopically. Usually only the anterior tips of the ciliary ridges are exposed even with scleral indentation, precluding treatment of the entire process. Nevertheless the procedure which is easy and relatively safe, may be useful in some patients in avoiding or delaying major surgery. Patients must be followed closely after laser treatment.

► Shields et al. present results that reveal transpupillary argon laser cyclophotocoagulation of the ciliary processes to be an archaic procedure with a low success rate and a moderately high rate of complications. Although in the discussion they describe the possibilities of the procedure as favorably as possible, clearly it cannot compete on any front with thermal neodymium: yttrium/aluminum/garnet laser transscleral cyclophotocoagulation using noncontact (Lasag) or contact (Surgical Laser Technologies) techniques for cyclodestruction.—R.P. Wilson, M.D.

## Long-Term Reduction of Intraocular Pressure After Repeat Argon Laser Trabeculoplasty

Grayson DK, Camras CB, Podos SM, Lustgarten JS (Mt Sinai School of Medicine, New York)
*Am J Ophthalmol* 106:312–321, September 1988                                    3–7

It is not clear whether argon laser trabeculoplasty negates the need for filtering surgery or merely postpones it. Thirty-eight eyes in 31 patients with glaucoma that responded to initial argon laser trabeculoplasty required a repeated procedure after a mean of nearly 2 years because of inadequate pressure control. A mean of 65 burns were placed initially, and 58 at the repeated procedure.

One eye underwent filtering surgery within 3 months of the first repeated laser trabeculoplasty, whereas 78% of eyes were considered to have responded. Two of 30 eyes observed for 1 year underwent filtering surgery, and three had a second repeat trabeculoplasty. On follow-up for a mean of 21 months, 15 eyes underwent a second repeated laser procedure; 7 of these eyes later required filtering surgery.

A smaller number of initial burns may relate to successful repeated laser trabeculoplasty in patients with glaucoma. It remains unclear how either the argon or the neodymium: yttrium/aluminum/garnet laser reduces intraocular pressure. Repeated laser trabeculoplasty should be strongly considered in patients who benefit from an initial procedure. In some cases the intraocular pressure may remain low for longer than 2 years. Many patients, however, will eventually require filtering surgery after a third laser trabeculoplasty.

▶ Long-term experience with argon laser trabeculoplasty (ALT) has shown it to be a time-limited procedure, secondary to either the ongoing disease process or waning tissue effects. This study shows that repeated ALT can be successful, although accompanied by greater risk. The limited number of burns per full treatment in this study is closer to the standard 180-degree treatment than the Wise protocol of 100 burns over 360 degrees. This undoubtedly accounts for their success rate on repeating the procedure a second time. My indications include (1) history of a good result from a properly applied ALT; (2) at least a year's lapse since the previous procedure; and (3) intraocular pressure such as a 25% drop will result in satisfactory pressure control. If 100 burns have been used each session, I do not repeat the procedure more than once.—R.P. Wilson, M.D.

---

## A Complication From Alcohol-Swabbed Tonometer Tips

Soukiasian SH, Asdourian GK, Weiss JS, Kachadoorian HA (Univ of Massachusetts, Worcester)
*Am J Ophthalmol* 105:424–425, April 1988                                            3–8

It has been proposed that tonometer tips be disinfected with 70% isopropyl alcohol wipes to prevent transmission of viruses. However, in a woman aged 38 years with type I diabetes, corneal epithelial opacification developed corresponding to the area of the tonometer tip. The area stained faintly with fluorescein and strongly with rose bengal. Discomfort lasted for several hours after a 2-hour period of patching. A similar effect was noted in a second patient undergoing tonometry, but it was less marked.

Isolation of human immunodeficiency virus from the tears of AIDS patients, as well as isolation of herpes simplex virus (HSV) type 1, hepatitis B virus, and adenovirus, have raised concern over iatrogenic transmission by the ophthalmologist. Swabbing the tonometer tip with a 70% isopropyl alcohol wipe is effective against HSV 1 and adenovirus, and it is practical and convenient. A delay of 1 minute after disinfecting the tonometer tip prevents side effects. Alternately, the tip could be swabbed immediately after each use.

▶ The acquired immunodeficiency syndrome epidemic has heightened the awareness of physician and patient alike to the possibility of infectious disease transmission with tonometry. The ophthalmologist, however, cannot forget that solutions toxic to viruses are also toxic to the corneal epithelium. Attention to practice routine is necessary to prevent complications.—R.P. Wilson, M.D.

**Long-Term Betaxolol Therapy in Glaucoma Patient With Pulmonary Disease**
Weinreb RN, van Buskirk EM, Cherniack R, Drake MM (Univ of California, San Diego; Univ of Oregon; Health Science Ctr, Portland; Natl Jewish Ctr for Immunology and Respiratory Medicine, Denver; Alcon Labs, Inc, Fort Worth. Texas)
*Am J Ophthalmol* 106:162–167, August 1988                                    3–9

Bronchoconstriction may develop in susceptible patients with lung disease given systemic or topical β blockers. The cardioselective β blocker betaxolol was evaluated in 101 patients with glaucoma who had chronic obstructive lung disease, asthma, or bronchoconstriction related to timolol administration. A 0.5% betaxolol preparation was given twice daily, and patients were examined every 3 months for up to 2 years.

Initially, the ratio of forced expiratory volume in 1 second (FEV$_1$) to forced vital capacity (FVC) was 66%. After 2 weeks of treatment with betaxolol the mean ratio of FEV$_1$/FVC was still 66%, and after 1 year it was 60%; at 2 years the ratio declined to 54%. Nine patients withdrew from the study because of symptoms possibly associated with betaxolol therapy; 5 of them had symptomatic pulmonary obstruction.

Several clinical studies indicate that betaxolol is safer than the nonselective β blocker timolol in patients with coexisting pulmonary disease. Although not all patients with glaucoma tolerate betaxolol, most of those with lung disease can safely receive this drug. Serial lung function assessment can help identify those patients in whom a cardioselective drug is appropriate.

▶ Patients with chronic obstructive pulmonary disease do better with betaxolol than patients with asthma do. My guidelines for the use of betaxolol in these patients include the following: (1) Topical miotics and epinephrine have already been used if tolerated. (2) The patient cannot be given antibronchospastic medication. (3) There is no history of a severe attack. Punctal occlusion is mandatory, and consultation with the patient's physician is suggested unless the disease is mild. If the severity of glaucoma makes the use of betaxolol attractive despite the risk, it is helpful to check the FEV$_1$/FVC ratio both before and after therapy.—R.P. Wilson, M.D.

**Topical β-Blocker Therapy and Central Nervous System Side Effects: A Preliminary Study Comparing Betaxolol and Timolol**
Lynch MG, Whitson JT, Brown RH, Nguyen H, Drake MM (Univ of Texas Southwestern Med Ctr, Dallas; Alcon Labs, Fort Worth)
*Arch Ophthalmol* 106:908–911, July 1988                                    3–10

Both systemic and topical β-blocker treatment may be associated with central nervous system (CNS) side effects such as sleep disorder, depression, and hallucinations. It is not clear whether selective β blockade is advantageous. Medication in 18 patients having CNS symptoms during

Symptoms Included in β-Blocker Questionnaire

| | |
|---|---|
| Irregular heartbeat | Poor appetite |
| High blood pressure | Abdominal pain |
| Difficulty breathing | Cramping |
| Wheezing | Nausea/vomiting |
| Fainting | Decreased taste |
| Depression | Tingling in fingers and toes |
| Mood swings (emotional lability) | General weakness or lethargy |
| Decreased sexual drive | Stinging or burning in eye |
| Impotence | Diarrhea |
| Rashes | Difficulty sleeping |

(Courtesy of Lynch MG, Whitson JT, Brown RH, et al: *Arch Ophthalmol* 106:908–911, July 1988.)

timolol therapy (table) was changed to 0.5% betaxolol twice daily. In a double-masked, crossover study, timolol was discontinued in 7 patients with symptoms; these patients were then assigned to receive either 0.5% timolol or 0.5% betaxolol.

In the open-label trial, the most frequent side effects were depression and emotional lability. Sixteen of 18 patients improved when given betaxolol in place of timolol. In the double-masked study, 5 of 7 patients improved subjectively when using betaxolol rather than timolol.

There may be some advantage in using a selective rather than a nonselective β blocker. Patients experiencing CNS side effects from timolol therapy may improve if betaxolol is substituted.

▶ This article is somewhat understated as betaxolol is definitely a safer drug causing fewer systemic side effects, whether they be pulmonary, cardiac, or CNS in nature. The reader should see the original article if he is interested in why a cardioselective β blocker has less effect on the heart than a nonselective agent. The other side of the coin is that betaxolol is less effective, sometimes significantly.—R.P. Wilson, M.D.

## Long-Term Evaluation of 0.25% Levobunolol and Timolol for Therapy for Elevated Intraocular Pressure

Boozman FW III, Carriker R, Foerster R, Allen RC, Novack GD, Batoosingh AL (Univ of Virginia, Charlottesville; Univ of California, Irvine; Allergan Inc, Irving, Calif)

*Arch Ophthalmol* 106:614–618, May 1988                                                     3–11

Although 0.5% timolol maleate is most often used to lower elevated intraocular pressure (IOP), a 0.25% preparation may be equally effective. A 1-year double-masked study was carried out to compare twice-daily treatment with 0.25% timolol maleate or levobunolol in 78 patients having glaucoma or ocular hypertension. When necessary, the concentration of medication was increased to 0.5%; patients were then followed for another 3 months.

The mean IOP declined by 4.6 mm Hg with timolol and by 5.1 mm Hg with levobunolol. Twenty-nine of 41 patients receiving timolol and 26 of

37 receiving levobunolol successfully completed the first phase of the study. Of those requiring 0.5% medication, 8 of 11 taking timolol and 3 of 4 taking levobunolol successfully completed the second phase. The higher concentration did produce a slightly greater reduction in IOP. Side effects were comparable with both medications.

Twice daily treatment with 0.25% timolol or levobunolol is an effective means of lowering elevated IOP. There was little evidence of tolerance to either medication. Previous long-term studies have shown little difference between 0.25% and 0.5% concentrations of these drugs. If pressure is not controlled, however, the 0.5% preparation might be tried before other medications are added.

▶ Boozman et al. again show that there is very little difference in effect or length of action between the 0.25% and 0.5% strengths of nonselective β blockers. With the known list of serious side effects of these agents continuing to grow, it is prudent to use the least effective dosage. At this time, that would be timolol 0.25% once or twice a day, or levobunolol 0.5%, daily, both with light lid closure or punctal occlusion, or both.—R.P. Wilson, M.D.

---

**Effect of Changing Medication Regimens in Glaucoma Patients**
Novack GD, David R, Lee PF, Freeman MI, Duzman E, Batoosingh AL (Univ of California, Irvine; Ben-Gurion Univ, Beer-Sheva, Israel; Albany Med College, NY; Virginia Mason Clinic, Seattle)
*Ophthalmologica* 196:23–28, 1988                                           3–12

---

When current glaucoma medication fails to control the intraocular pressure adequately, a second drug often is added. The authors studied the effect of changing to another β blocker before adding a second drug to the regimen of patients who have no response to 0.5% timolol. The alternative drug was 0.5% or 1.0% levobunolol. In addition, the effect of study participation on compliance was assessed in control patients continuing to take 0.5% timolol therapy. Thirty patients received levobunolol and 13 received timolol. Sixteen of the 43 patients completed the 3-month study.

From 30% to 40% of patients in each treatment group had successful control of the intraocular pressure throughout the 3-month study period. The others did not have significant pressure reductions and were withdrawn from the study within 2 weeks. One third of the patients continuing to take timolol responded adequately, despite previous failure of this treatment. Improved patient compliance apparently had a major role.

Careful interpretation is necessary of the results of "switch" studies that lack a control group. Initiation of a "new" regimen with an equally effective β blocker may increase patient compliance and thereby control intraocular pressure adequately in those who have seemingly failed to respond to initial treatment.

▶ This study shows that there is little, if any, benefit in switching between nonselective β blockers if the first does not control intraocular pressure adequately. It does reveal that increased attention to the patient and his or her cooperation with treatment can often yield remarkable improvement in the effectiveness of any regimen.—R.P. Wilson, M.D.

## Aphakic Cystoid Macular Edema Secondary to Betaxolol Therapy
Hesse RJ, Swan JL II (Ochsner Clin and Alton Ochsner Med Found, New Orleans)
*Ophthalmic Surg* 19:562–564, August 1988                    3–13

Topical epinephrine can lead to cystoid macular edema after surgery to treat aphakic glaucoma. A similar response to betaxolol, a drug that preferentially blocks $\beta_1$ receptors, was observed.

Woman, *85*, underwent bilateral intracapsular cataract extraction. When examined 6 years later she had an acuity of 20/40 bilaterally with aphakic correction. Sector iridectomies and ruptured anterior hyaloids were present in both eyes. Subsequently, the intraocular pressure rose in the right eye, and 0.5% betaxolol was used in both eyes on a twice-daily basis. Fluctuating blurred vision ensued, with markedly reduced acuity. Fluorescein angiography showed marked cystoid macular edema in both eyes. Vision improved after betaxolol was withdrawn, and the macular edema resolved substantially. It recurred in the right eye when betaxolol was resumed and again resolved when the drug was discontinued. Most recently, acuity was 20/50 in the right eye and 20/40 in the left.

The constitution of adrenergic receptors in a given patient determines the pharmacologic response to an adrenergic agent. $\beta$ Blockers may exhibit paradoxic adrenergic stimulation, as in this patient, in whom betaxolol therapy was associated with aphakic cystoid macular edema.

▶ Forewarned is forearmed. I would not let this report dissuade me from using $\beta$ blockers when needed in surgical aphakia. However, if the patient complains of compromised vision, cystoid macular edema should be considered in the differential diagnosis.—R.P. Wilson, M.D.

## Antiglaucoma Therapy During Pregnancy: Parts I and II
Kooner KS, Zimmerman TJ (Louisiana State Univ, Shreveport; Univ of Louisville)
*Ann Ophthalmol* 20:166–169, 208, May 1988                    3–14

Problems arise if a glaucoma patient receiving treatment becomes pregnant, or if glaucoma develops in a pregnant woman. Toxic effects on both the mother and fetus may be taken into account. All ophthalmic topical medications should be considered to produce systemic blood levels. Although teratogenic effects are possible, it seldom is feasible to specify a causal relationship between a specific drug and an adverse pregnancy outcome.

Drugs given to the mother may cross the placenta and affect the fetus or appear in breast milk. Alpha-fetoproteins may interfere with normal drug-binding processes. Lipid-soluble, nonionized, low-molecular-weight drugs readily cross the placenta. Once a drug enters the fetal circulation, it may be excreted into amniotic fluid from the kidneys, lungs, or skin. Lipid-soluble drugs of low molecular weight most readily enter breast milk, but more than 1% to 2% of the adminstered dose rarely is secreted into the milk.

The first trimester is the critical period for teratogenic drug effects. The central nervous system and the endocrine, genital, and immune systems develop further in the second and third trimesters. Once the placenta is detached, any drug retained by the neonate may not be properly metabolized because of immature hepatic and renal function.

If drug treatment of a pregnant patient is necessary, a minimal effective dose should be given for as short a time as possible. Nasolacrimal occlusion limits systemic absorption after instilling an ocular medication. Patients should be advised not to breast-feed their infants. Laser therapy may be considered as an alternative to medication. Causal relationships between drug treatment in pregnancy and teratogenic changes should be viewed cautiously unless the association is highly convincing.

▶ The use of glaucoma medications during pregnancy is a soul-searching decision for the physician and patient. This editorial, although having few studies to go on, provides the best review to date. Dipivefrin in its active form is an endogenous hormone in low concentrations and is my choice in most situations.— R.P. Wilson, M.D.

---

**Evaluation of the T Test as a Method of Detecting Visual Field Changes**
Hills JF, Johnson CA (Univ of California, Davis)
*Ophthalmology* 95:261–266, February 1988                    3–15

---

Comparisons of sequential visual field records are necessary to assess the progression or resolution of ocular anomalies and to evaluate treatments. Quantitative automated perimetry offers a simple means of objectively studying visual field changes in various clinical settings. The paired comparison *t* test has been used to compare sensitivity differences between 2 sets of visual field data. The Delta program for the Octopus perimeter uses a *t* test to provide an objective comparison of visual fields.

Computer simulations generated pairs of visual fields with known alterations, and these were compared by the *t* test procedure. An initial field based on normal data was compared with the same data after a scotoma of known size and depth was introduced. The *t* test proved sensitive to small changes of the entire visual field, such as those produced by variations in day-to-day sensitivity and changes in pupil size. However, the *t* test did not reliably detect scotomas of 18 degrees or less in diameter, even when the loss of sensitivity exceeded 35 dB.

The paired comparison *t* test, although sensitive to small differential changes in the full visual field and hemifield, is insensitive to small to moderate scotomata. Scotomata involving 1 or 2 test locations are not detected regardless of the density of the defect. The test does not take into account the spatial relation of test sites exhibiting sensitivity loss. The clinical usefulness of the paired comparison *t* test, therefore, is limited.

▶ Hills and Johnson correctly point out how inaccurate the Delta program of the Octopus is in determining progression. The most realistic use for the Delta program is to show the difference in sensitivity (change mode) at each locus between 2 fields. The responsibility remains with the ophthalmologist to interpret the results.—R.P. Wilson, M.D.

---

**Reliability Indexes of Automated Perimetric Tests**
Katz J, Sommer A (Wilmer Inst, Johns Hopkins Med Insts)
*Arch Ophthalmol* 106:1252–1254, September 1988                    3–16

---

Many automated perimeters have standardized algorithms for evaluating the reliability of test results. Because the test is not adjusted, the clinician must interpret "unreliable" results cautiously. The Humphrey Visual Field Analyzer provides 3 measures of test reliability: the proportion of fixation losses and the false positive and false negative responses. Tests on up to 40% of glaucomatous eyes and 23% of normal eyes have been considered unreliable.

Reliability criteria were examined in 76 glaucoma patients and 248 normal controls who had visual field testing with the Humphrey device. Forty-five percent of results in glaucoma patients and 30% of those in controls were considered unreliable according to the manufacturer's criteria because most of them failed to meet the criterion for fixation loss. The higher rejection rate in glaucoma patients reflected their higher rate of false negative responses. The difference did not relate to factors such as age, pupil diameter, or visual acuity.

Patients with high false positive rates often have high rates of fixation loss. It may help to interrupt the test and reinstruct the patient. The blind spot may be misplaced initially or the patient may fail to fixate or respond to motor noise. The higher false negative response rate in glaucoma patients may be because of increased visual fatigue and variability early in the disease.

Decisions on glaucoma status should not be based solely on the results of any single automated visual field test. If fixation loss remains a problem in follow-up studies with the Humphrey device, the 20% fixation loss cutoff may have to be reassessed.

---

**A Comparison of the Blue Color Mechanism in High- and Low-Tension Glaucoma**
Yamazaki Y, Lakowski R, Drance SM (Univ of British Columbia, Vancouver)
*Ophthalmology* 96:12–15, January 1989                    3–17

---

Some glaucoma suspects have impaired color discrimination, especially in the blue-yellow or blue-green spectrum measured at the fovea. However, some eyes with advanced glaucomatous field defects have normal color scores. Spectral increment thresholds were compared in 25 patients with low-tension glaucoma and 25 with high-tension glaucoma, who had similar degrees of visual field loss.

Patients with high-tension glaucoma had significantly increased chromatic thresholds compared with those having low-tension glaucoma. The differences were greatest in the blue color range. Mean achromatic thresholds also were significantly increased in patients with high-tension glaucoma, except in the short wavelength range.

In high-tension glaucoma there are significant losses in both chromatic and achromatic spectral sensitivities at all wavelengths. Some patients, however, have normal thresholds similar to those in patients with low-tension glaucoma. Blue chromatic and achromatic signals travel in larger-diameter axons than those processing red-green information, and larger fibers are more vulnerable to increased pressure. The findings support the view that different mechanisms of damage may operate in the glaucomas.

## Age-Related Loss of Morphologic Responses to Pilocarpine in Rhesus Monkey Ciliary Muscle

Lütjen-Drecoll E, Tamm E, Kaufman PL (Univ of Erlangen-Nürnberg, Erlangen, West Germany; Univ of Wisconsin)
*Arch Ophthalmol* 106:1591–1598, November 1988                     3–18

Earlier studies suggested that lenticular factors rather than decreased ciliary muscle contractility were involved in presbyopia. This assumption was reassessed in the rhesus monkey, which has an accommodative apparatus similar to that in humans. Morphological and topographic ciliary muscle responses to pilocarpine and atropine were studied at various ages.

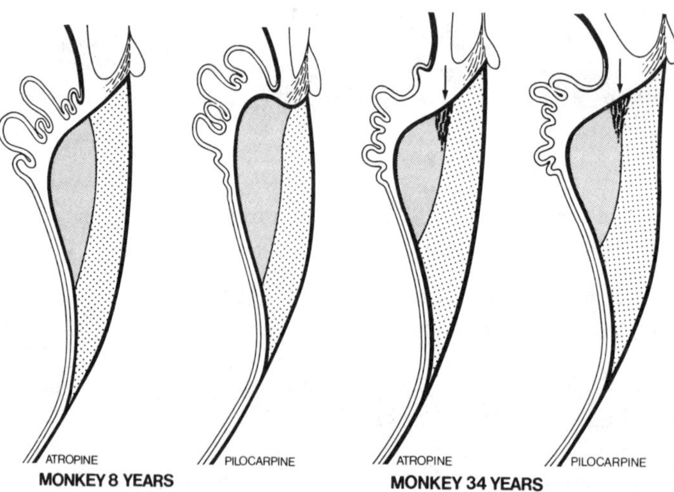


**Fig 3–2.**—Ciliary muscle topography and connective tissue distribution in rhesus monkeys. Representative sections are depicted schematically. **Left,** 8-year-old rhesus monkey has essentially no intramuscular connective tissue. **Right,** 34-year-old rhesus monkey has connective tissue *(arrows)* only anteriorly between longitudinal and reticular zones. (Courtesy of Lütjen-Drecoll E, Tamm E, Kaufman PL: *Arch Ophthalmol* 106:1591–1598, November 1988.)

Although the general shape of the ciliary muscle and the size of its subdivisions were similar at all ages, the connective tissue ground plate between the muscle and the ciliary processes thickened with advancing age (Fig 3–2). Atropinized muscle became shorter and smaller in area with age. Contractile responses to pilocarpine declined in older animals at a rate similar to that of the accommodative decrease.

Forward movement of the lens depends on anterointernal movement of the zonular attachment to the valleys of the pars plicata ciliary processes. The aged ciliary muscle becomes unresponsive to pilocarpine. The increase in connective tissue seems too small to immobilize the muscle. Another possibility is that muscle or nerve fibers are altered or lost. The present findings direct attention away from the lens and toward pathophysiology of the ciliary muscle in presbyopia.

## Glaucoma in Patients With Ocular Cicatricial Pemphigoid
Tauber J, Melamed S, Foster CS (Massachusetts Eye and Ear Infirmary, Boston; Harvard Med School)
*Ophthalmology* 96:33–37, January 1989                                    3–19

Cicatricial pemphigoid (CP) is a systemic autoimmune disorder characterized by conjunctival scarring and eventual corneal opacification and marked visual loss. The eye may be totally lost. Up to a third of patients with CP may have ocular hypertension or glaucoma. Glaucoma was found in 26% of 111 patients with ocular CP. Most of them had advanced glaucoma, and this was associated with high-grade conjunctival inflammation. Twenty-seven of the 29 affected patients had a history of glaucoma for a mean of 11.3 years before CP was di-agnosed.

Genetic explanations for the prevalence of glaucoma in CP are largely speculative. It is possible that the explanation lies in drug-induced cicatricial changes, because a long history of glaucoma and chronic medication use are the rule. Extraocular manifestations of CP occur in one fifth of patients, indicating a systemic, presumably autoimmune disease.

Patients with CP should be followed closely for glaucoma. Laser trabeculoplasty may be difficult in these cases. The question of whether to continue topical antiglaucoma medications is unresolved, but a drug holiday may be informative. More aggressive approaches to controlling intraocular pressure should be considered in patients with CP. These include cyclocryotherapy, transscleral laser cyclophotocoagulation, and even placement of an aqueous shunting device.

## The Presentation and Prognosis of Glaucoma in Pseudoexfoliation of the Lens Capsule
Brooks AMV, Gillies WE (The Royal Victorian Eye and Ear Hosp, East Melbourne, Victoria, Australia)
*Ophthalmology* 95:271–276, February 1988                                    3–20

Too little is known about the prognosis in pseudoexfoliation (PXF) of the lens capsule, unless both elevated intraocular pressure (IOP) and field loss are present at the outset. Data were reviewed on 519 patients with PXF; 286 of them had glaucoma. Most had chronic open-angle glaucoma, but 65 patients had acute glaucoma.

In unilateral PXF glaucoma, the presence of PXF in the fellow eye was a serious risk factor. The IOP became elevated in nearly three fourths of these eyes, and nearly one fourth became glaucomatous during a 6-year mean follow-up. During this same period, glaucoma developed in one fourth of eyes with ocular hypertension at presentation. When the IOP was normal initially, increased pressure developed in only 1 of 8 eyes and glaucoma developed in one third of these eyes. Open-angle PXF glaucoma in acute cases usually responded well to medical treatment initially, but failure frequently ensued. Laser trabeculoplasty often succeeded in conjunction with medical treatment. Surgery often was necessary and usually was effective, although adjuvant medical therapy was often needed.

Ocular hypertension should be treated medically in patients with PXF syndrome. Patients with normal IOP initially can be followed up regularly. Glaucoma in PXF usually is a secondary form. Early surgery should be considered once cupping and field loss are present if there is difficulty in controlling the pressure medically especially if the other eye has responded well to surgery.

▶ Interesting aspects of this study include the low incidence of glaucoma development (5 of 134 eyes) during a 6-year period in patients with PXF but with normal IOP and the high frequency of failure with medical therapy that was initially successful. These findings suggest a less dire stance in dealing with PXF patients without ocular hypertension and a more aggressive approach in dealing with patients with borderline IOP control on medical therapy.—R.P. Wilson, M.D.

---

## Intraocular Pressure Effects of Carbonic Anhydrase Inhibitors in Primary Open-Angle Glaucoma

Lichter PR, Musch DC, Medzihradsky F, Standardi CL (Univ of Michigan)
*Am J Ophthalmol* 107:11–17, January 1989                    3–21

---

Three commonly used oral carbonic anhydrase inhibitors—acetazolamide tablets, acetazolamide Sequels, and methazolamide tablets—were evaluated in a randomized study of 19 patients with confirmed primary open-angle glaucoma. Average peak reductions in intraocular pressure were compared and a statistical modeling approach also was used.

Each preparation was more effective in lowering intraocular patient when given to a patient who already had received the preparation. A dose-response effect was seen with both acetazolamide preparations. A 500-mg dose of acetazolamide tablets rapidly reduced the intraocular pressure.

Acetazolamide appears to have a greater initial effect on intraocular pressure than methazolamide in patients with primary open-angle glaucoma. When intraocular pressure must be rapidly reduced, the use of 500 mg of acetazolamide tablets is recommended. Intravenous administration probably would be even more effective. Combining a carbonic anhydrase inhibitor with a β blocker should be considered. The optimal dose of carbonic anhydrase inhibitor for chronic use is still not known.

---

**Juvenile Glaucoma, Race, and Refraction**
Lotufo D, Ritch R, Szmyd L Jr, Burris JE (New York Eye and Ear Infirmary)
*JAMA* 261:249–252, Jan 13, 1989                               3–22

---

Juvenile glaucoma encompasses all forms of glaucoma in patients aged 10–35 years. The visual outcome is worse for younger patients with glaucoma, but the factors disposing to increased intraocular pressure or glaucomatous damage are not well understood.

A series of 244 consecutive patients aged 10–35 years were seen from 1984 to 1986, among them, 25 with juvenile ocular hypertension and 43 with juvenile primary open-angle glaucoma. Blacks constituted 47% of the patients with primary open-angle glaucoma and 20% of ocular hypertensives. In both groups blacks presented at younger ages than whites. Myopia was present in 59% of the ocular hypertensives and in 73% of patients with open-angle glaucoma. All eyes of black patients with more than 3D of myopia and half of such eyes in whites had glaucomatous defects.

Myopia is closely associated with juvenile open-angle glaucoma. Young blacks with elevated intraocular pressure—especially those who are myopic—are more susceptible than whites to glaucomatous damage. Intraocular pressure should be measured as a routine part of the eye examination in patients of all ages. Blacks should have tonometry periodically, especially if they are myopic.

# 4 Neuro-Ophthalmology

---

## Is Neuro-Ophthalmology Becoming Interventional?

ROBERT C. SERGOTT, M.D.
*Neuro-Ophthalmology Service, Wills Eye Hospital, Philadelphia, Pennsylvania*

Ever since Llewellyn Paton detected chiasmal mass lesions for Harvey Cushing with tangent screen visual field examinations, neuro-ophthalmologists have been the prototype "rainmakers" for neurosurgery. This role has been expanded to include detection of lesions for other surgical colleagues including otolaryngologists and orbital surgeons.

Neuro-ophthalmologists, in general, have been regarded as a somewhat obtuse, hybrid breed, linking the enigmas of the central nervous system with the precise technology of ophthalmology. In the past, they enthralled their ophthalmic, neurologic, and neurosurgical colleagues by discovering massive tumors and aneurysms that presented with the most minimal of physical findings.

However, in the mid-1970s with the advent of computed tomographic (CT) scanning, neuro-ophthalmology changed forever. First CT scanning, and more recently magnetic resonance imaging (MRI) scanning, permit even the most disinterested clinician a direct view into the orbit, chiasm, and entire central nervous system. Neuro-ophthalmologists realized that their practices were changing greatly several years ago when it became the fashionable statement to portray our practices as consisting of "CT and MRI negative diseases."

More precise neuro-imaging procedures, however, may not represent the gallows for neuro-ophthalmology, but may be the catalyst to move neuro-ophthalmologists into an "interventional realm." Just as, several years ago, neuro-radiology developed a special field of "interventional neuro-radiology" consisting of angiographers who were bold enough to consider treating any lesion within reach of their catheter, so 1988 witnessed a similar change in the perspective of the neuro-ophthalmic literature. Many excellent papers are still written concerning new, valuable clinical observations, but a new philosophy of neuro-ophthalmic treatment seems to be arising with promise and determination.

The optic neuritis treatment trial (ONTT) is being chaired by Dr. Roy Beck of the University of South Florida, and this 14-center study for the first time is examining in a clinical, scientific way the therapeutic interventions for one of the most common neuro-ophthalmic disorders.

In an even more therapeutically aggressive stance, Dr. Hanneken and coworkers at the Wilmer Ophthalmological Institute at Johns Hopkins have joined forces with the neurosurgeons and neuroradiologists to approach engorged superior ophthalmic veins through the orbit to successfully eradicate potentially blinding and disfiguring vascular malformations in the cavernous sinus (1).

Finally, neuro-ophthalmologists have recaptured the therapy of chronic papilledema secondary to pseudotumor cerebri from the neurologists and neuro-surgeons (2–5). It appears as though never again will neuro-ophthalmologists merely diagnose pseudotumor cerebri, treat with diuretics or corticosteroids, and then shunt the patients over to the neurosurgeons for a variety of cerebrospinal fluid diversion procedures. In what amounts to an unplanned, multicenter study of optic nerve sheath decompression in pseudotumor cerebri, five different surgeons, performing essentially the same operation, have established that optic nerve sheath decompression, when performed by experienced neuro-ophthalmic surgeons, may be the treatment of choice for vision threatening papilledema. Dr. John Keltner, of the University of California at Davis, has written in an accompanying editorial that "these results confirm that optic nerve decompression can be effective on a long term basis" (2).

Therefore, neuro-ophthalmology is a discipline in transition. These subspecialists who once only drew visual fields to guide their neurosurgical colleagues to the site of pathology have now moved into an exciting new era. They have shown that the optic nerve is a surgically accessible structure and since it may now be reached safely there is the potential to intervene in many other disorders. However, this potential for intervention holds within it a chance for surgical abuse, and therefore neuro-ophthalmologists have a tremendous responsibility to carry out these potential investigations in a cautious, disciplined manner. The promise is great, the opportunity abounds, yet the enthusiasm must be controlled.

*References*

1. Hanneken AM, Miller NR, Debrund GM, et al: Treatment of carotid-cavernous sinus fistulas using a detachable balloon catheter through the superior ophthalmic vein. *Arch Ophthalmol* 107:87–92, 1989.
2. Keltner JR: Optic nerve sheath decompression: How does it work?: Has its time come? *Arch Ophthalmol* 106:1365–1369, 1988.
3. Brourman ND, Spoor TC, Ramocki JM: Optic nerve sheath decompression for pseudotumor cerebri. *Arch Ophthalmol* 106:1378–1383, 1988.
4. Sergott RC, Savino PJ, Bosley TM: Modified optic nerve sheath decompression provides long term visual improvement for pseudotumor cerebri. *Arch Ophthalmol* 106:1384–1390, 1988.
5. Corbett JJ, Nerad JA, Zee DT, et al: Results of optic nerve sheath fenestration for pseudotumor cerebri. *Arch Ophthalmol* 106:1391–1397, 1988.

---

**Low-Contrast Letter Charts to Detect Subtle Neuropathies**
Drucker MD, Savino PJ, Sergott RC, Bosley TM, Schatz NJ, Kubilis PS (Wills Eye Hosp, Philadelphia; Fred Hutchinson Cancer Research Ctr, Seattle)
*Am J Ophthalmol* 105:141–145, February 1988                     4–1

Detection of visual contrast sensitivity loss is important in the early recognition of undiagnosed optic neuropathies. An affected patient may have normal Snellen acuity and visual impairment only under low-contrast conditions. The value of Regan charts in detecting subtle optic nerve dysfunction was studied in 31 patients with neuropathy and a Snellen acuity of at least 20/30 in the involved eye. Regan contrast chart testing was carried out using a standard Snellen acuity chart with 95% contrast between the darker optotypes and lighter background and one using Snellen optotypes with only a 9% contrast differential. Normal values were determined in 20 controls.

One half of the 35 eyes with optic neuropathy had a decrease in correct responses on Ishihara color plates. Twenty-four of the 31 patients had an afferent detect. The Regan low-contrast letter charts were 93% sensitive in detecting optic neuropathy. Correlation between Regan chart values and color vision testing was poor.

The Regan low-contrast letter charts can identify patients having dysfunction as well as normal persons with high accuracy. In such states as glaucoma, cataract, retinal disease, and optic neuropathy, discrimination of low-contrast objects may be reduced while detection of high-contrast optotypes is relatively spared. Symmetrical optic neuropathies are readily detected using the Regan charts. The test is inexpensive, test time is short, and paramedical personnel can administer it.

▶ The ophthalmologist must not just check vision but also evaluate the entire afferent system. These charts are an inexpensive, reliable, quick method to localize difficult and unusual visual symptoms and are much more cost efficient and safer than scanning with computed tomography or magnetic resonance imaging.—R.C. Sergott, M.D.

## Uremic Optic Neuropathy

Knox DL, Hanneken AM, Hollows FC, Miller NR, Schick HL Jr, Gonzales WL (Wilmer Ophthalmological Inst, Baltimore; Univ of New South Wales, Kensington, Australia)
*Arch Ophthalmol* 106:50–54, January 1988

4–2

Six patients with severe renal disease had progressive visual loss, decreased pupillary reactions to light, and optic nerve swelling. The patients were uremic and anemic, and 4 had moderately or severely elevated blood pressure. Visual loss occurred relatively rapidly after several days or weeks of blurred vision. Acuity ranged from no light perception to 20/60. Four patients had marked optic nerve head swelling. In 2 cases edema extended into the macula. Hemodialysis was followed by improved vision in 4 patients. Another patient improved when oral corticosteroid therapy was resumed. A patient with renal transplant rejection who had early cryptococcal meningitis did not recover vision.

Optic neuropathy apparently can complicate kidney disease and uremia. Patients may have severe optic neuropathy and edema extending into the retina, optic atrophy without visible swelling of the disk, or moderately severe retinal edema extending into the macula. The disorder calls for prompt hemodialysis and cranial computed tomography to rule out mass lesions and hydrocephalus. Antihypertensive therapy is given if the blood pressure is elevated. Oral corticosteroid therapy may be indicated in addition to dialysis. If a renal transplant is being rejected, lumbar puncture is done to rule out cryptococcal meningitis.

▶ Visual loss caused by optic nerve disease always demands aggressive management to identify treatable disorders. In patients with renal failure after infections and mass lesions have been excluded in evaluation of a new optic neuropathy, clinicians should institute aggressive hemodialysis in an attempt to restore vision.—R.C. Sergott, M.D.

**Optic Gliomas: A Reanalysis of the University of California, San Francisco Experience**
Wong JYC, Uhl V, Wara WM, Sheline GE (Univ of California, San Francisco)
*Cancer* 60:1847–1855, Oct 15, 1987                                                                4–3

The best management of optic gliomas remains uncertain, but most reports indicate that they are not self-limited tumors. Twenty-four of 38 patients seen from 1953 to 1984 underwent megavoltage radiotherapy. Eight patients, all younger than 10 years, had stigmata of neurofibromatosis. Twenty-seven patients had tumor biopsy, and 3 others underwent exploratory craniotomy. Twenty chiasmal tumors and 4 optic nerve tumors received a mean dose of 4,800 cGY. The mean follow-up was 9.4 years.

One of 4 irradiated patients with optic nerve tumors failed to respond and was salvaged by surgery. Treatment in only 9 of 20 irradiated patients with chiasmal tumors failed, compared with 6 of 7 unirradiated patients. Overall actuarial survival at 10 years was 87%, and the relapse-free survival rate was 55%. Chiasmal gliomas carried a poorer prognosis than optic nerve tumors, independent of invasion into adjacent brain tissue. Among patients with chiasmal tumors, those older than 20 years of age had a worse outlook. In only 1 of 5 nonirradiated patients with optic nerve tumors did treatment fail.

Optic nerve gliomas carry a relatively good prognosis of survival, whereas many patients with recurrent chiasmal tumors eventually die of disease. Radiotherapy appears to be helpful to patients with chiasmal glioma and can lead to improved vision and fewer relapses. A dose of 50–60 Gy to mature brain in 5–6.5 weeks is recommended. Tumors confined to 1 optic nerve may be resected.

▶ The biologic behavior of these neoplasms is more heterogeneous than once suspected. The ophthalmologist must not dismiss such lesions as only visual problems but realize that these tumors may endanger life. Prompt oncologic evaluation and frequent follow-up clinical and neuroradiologic monitoring are mandatory.—R.C. Sergott, M.D.

## Horner's Syndrome in Children

Woodruff G, Buncic JR, Morin JD (The Hosp for Sick Children, Toronto)
*J Pediatr Ophthalmol Strabismus* 25:40–44, January–February 1988      4–4

Ten children up to 8 years of age with Horner's syndrome underwent pharmacologic testing and computed tomography (CT). In addition, they were assessed for iris color and facial sweating.

None of the children had classic preganglionic Horner's syndrome associated with brachial plexus birth injury (table). Two patients had neuroblastoma. Both had ptosis and Horner's syndrome developed before age 1 year. Both patients with neuroblastoma had a preganglionic lesion, as indicated by anhidrosis and OH-amphetamine testing. These were the only patients having anhidrosis coinciding with preganglionic localization by hydroxyamphetamine. None of the 10 patients had heterochromia.

The onset of Horner's syndrome in a child may be a manifestation of neuroblastoma. An onset at birth or in childhood warrants investigation except when precipitated by thoracic surgery. The study should include a chest radiograph, CT of the head and neck, and a 24-hour urinary catecholamine assay.

▶ Clinical dogmas frequently need qualification and revision, and this article alerts clinicians to an important pediatric neuro-ophthalmic observation. Be-

Characteristics of 10 Children With Horner's Syndrome

| Case Number | Presentation | Localization by OH-Amphetamine | Anhydrosis | Diagnosis |
|---|---|---|---|---|
| 1 | Ptosis, 3rd & 6th nerve palsy at birth | Postganglionic | No | Arachnoidal cyst |
| 2 | Unequal sized pupils at birth | Preganglionic | No | No cause found |
| 3 | Ptosis at birth | Preganglionic | No | No cause found |
| 4 | Ptosis at birth | Preganglionic | Yes | Neuroblastoma |
| 5 | Long-standing at age 5 years | Preganglionic | No | Cerebral palsy (semilobar holoprosencephaly) |
| 6 | Acute febrile illness at age 7 months | Preganglionic | Yes | Neuroblastoma |
| 7 | Acute febrile illness at age 20 months | Preganglionic | No | No cause found |
| 8 | Ptosis at age 8 years | Preganglionic | No | No cause found |
| 9 | Surgery for coarctation of the aorta at age 5 years | Preganglionic | No | Cardiothoracic surgery |
| 10 | Surgery for tetralogy of Fallot at age 7 months | Preganglionic | No | Cardiothoracic surgery |

(Courtesy of Woodruff G, Buncic JR, Morin JD: *J Pediatr Ophthalmol Strabismus* 25:40–44, January–February 1988.)

cause in 2 patients in this series preganglionic Horner's syndrome was the first manifestation of neuroblastoma, thorough investigation of similar patients is warranted.—R.C. Sergott, M.D.

---

**Ocular Complications Associated With Retrobulbar Injections**
Morgan CM, Schatz H, Vine AK, Cantrill HL, Davidorf FH, Gitter KA, Rudich R (Univ of Michigan; Univ of California, San Francisco; Univ of Minnesota; Ohio State Univ; Retina Research Found, New Orleans; et al)
*Ophthalmology* 95:660–665, May 1988                                             4–5

---

Six complications of retrobulbar injection, documented in individual patients by fundus photography and fluorescein angiography, included steroid injection into the posterior ciliary artery circulation causing embolization of the choroid and optic nerve head, as well as ophthalmic artery injection of steroid, resulting in embolization of the choroidal and retinal circulations. In 1 patient lidocaine and air presumably were injected into the optic nerve sheath, extending anteriorly into the subretinal space. There also were findings of central retinal artery occlusion, partial injection of lidocaine into the central retinal artery with embolization of the retinal circulation, and presumed lidocaine injection into the optic nerve sheath, with combined central retinal vein and artery occlusion resulting.

Any unusual symptom such as marked pain or suddenly decreased acuity warrants immediate investigation. This is especially important when steroid or lidocaine is inadvertently injected intra-arterially. The optic nerve is in less danger when the globe is placed down and outward, rather than up and in. Peribulbar injection is an alternative to retrobulbar injection; a larger volume of anesthetic is injected through the lower lid with no attempt to enter the muscle cone. In retrobulbar injection, a 23-gauge blunt needle is used, and is advanced only as far as necessary to enter the muscle cone.

▶ This article documents potential complications of ophthalmic procedures under local anesthesia. Irreversible visual loss is possible, and patients need to be appraised of this rare occurrence when informed consent is obtained. Sudden pain or visual alteration mandates aggressive evaluation for this complication and consideration of maneuvers to lower intraocular pressure quickly. The risk of this rare complication may be the best argument to consider peribulbar anesthesia.—R.C. Sergott, M.D.

---

**Third Nerve Palsy and the Pupil: Footnotes to the Rule**
Trobe JD (Univ of Michigan)
*Arch Ophthalmol* 106:601–602, May 1988                                          4–6

---

Lustbader and Miller described a patient with isolated, pupil-sparing third nerve palsy and complete extraocular muscle paralysis caused by a basilar artery aneurysm. The case violated the Rule of the Pupil, which holds that when an aneurysm compresses the oculomotor nerve, the iris sphincter will be impaired, producing a dilated or sluggishly reactive pupil. The rule has held up quite well.

The rule is helpful in guiding decisions regarding angiography where noninvasive imaging is negative, but must be applied very cautiously to patients aged 20–50 years unless obvious vasculopathic risk factors are present. In addition, the rule is not applied if extraocular palsy is incomplete, and is applied cautiously to patients with complete oculomotor-innervated extraocular muscle palsy but only partial iris sphincter palsy. Patients with relative pupil sparing should not be grouped with those having absolute sparing. The rule should not be applied unless the third nerve palsy is isolated and there are no findings suggesting a noninfarctive cause.

▶ This editorial provides an insightful analysis of third nerve palsies, extracting a practical management approach from a large, and often confusing, literature. The busy clinician will serve his or her patients well to keep this article available for frequent review.—R.C. Sergott, M.D.

---

## Neurologic Disease in Biopsy-Proven Giant Cell (Temporal) Arteritis

Caselli RJ, Hunder GG, Whisnant JP (Mayo Clinic and Found, Rochester, Minn)
*Neurology* 38:352–359, March 1988                                         4–7

---

Neurologic findings were reviewed in 166 consecutive patients having biopsy-proved giant cell arteritis (128 women and 38 men with a median age at onset of 73 years). The median follow-up was 17 months.

Fifty-one patients (31%) had neurologic problems temporally related to giant cell arteritis (table). Thirty-five patients (21%) had ophthalmologic problems. A neuropathic syndrome was present in 23 patients, whereas 12 had transient ischemic attacks or brain infarction. Vertebrobasilar events were more frequent than in cerebral infarcts attributable to all causes. Eleven patients had neuro-otologic problems, most often vertigo. Five patients had a depressive syndrome. One patient had acute myelopathy. The most frequent ophthalmologic abnormalities were amaurosis fugax, permanent monocular visual loss without preceding amaurosis fugax, and scintillating scotoma.

Only 5 patients in this series had actual brain infarction; this may not significantly exceed the expected number in an age-matched population. Other neurologic disorders, however, are frequent in patients with active giant cell arteritis. About one fifth of patients in the present series had neuro-ophthalmologic problems.

▶ Whereas the major morbidity of giant cell arteritis remains permanent, irreversible blindness and other neurologic symptomatology should not necessarily be dismissed as "atherosclerotic" in nature. Ophthalmologists follow-

Neurologic Findings Related to Giant Cell Arteritis
in 51 Patients

| Finding | No. patients | (%) | Onset (mos)* |
|---|---|---|---|
| Neuropathic syndromes | 23 | (14) | +1 |
|   Mononeuropathies | 12 | (7) | +1 |
|   Peripheral neuropathy | 11 | (7) | 0 |
| TIA/brain infarction | 12 | (7) | +1 |
|   Carotid system | 8 | | |
|     TIA | 7 | | |
|     Infarct | 3 | | |
|   Vertebrobasilar system | 4 | | |
|     TIA | 3 | | |
|     Infarct | 2 | | |
| Neuro-otologic syndromes | 11 | (7) | +1 |
|   Isolated vertigo | 8 | | |
|   Vertigo and unilateral hearing loss | 1 | | |
|   Unilateral tinnitus | 2 | | |
| Tremor | 6 | (4) | +5 |
|   Essential | 2 | | |
|   Cerebellar | 3 | | |
|   Rest | 1 | | |
| Neuropsychiatric syndromes | 5 | (3) | −6 |
|   Organic affective disorder | 5 | | |
|   Dementia | 1 | | |
| Tongue numbness | 3 | (2) | +1 |
|   Unilateral | 2 | | |
|   Bilateral | 1 | | |
| Transverse myelopathy | 1 | (0.6) | 0 |

*+ = months after and − = months preceding temporal artery biopsy.
TIA = transient ischemic attack.
(Courtesy of Caselli RJ, Hunder GG, Whisnant JP: *Neurology* 38:352–359, March 1988.)

ing patients with giant cell arteritis should be alert to the possibility that new neurologic symptoms could herald a disease reactivation.—R.C. Sergott, M.D.

## Magnetic Resonance Imaging of the Optic Nerve in Optic Neuritis

Miller DH, Newton MR, van der Poel JC, du Boulay EPGH, Halliday AM, Kendall BE, Johnson G, MacManus DG, Moseley IF, McDonald WI (Inst of Neurology and National Hosps for Nervous Diseases, London)
*Neurology* 38:175–179, February 1988



Magnetic resonance (MR) imaging is a sensitive means of detecting lesions of multiple sclerosis (MS). Multifocal lesions are present in white matter in 90% or more of patients with clinically definite MS. Optic nerve abnormalities are detected using a short inversion time inversion recovery (STIR) sequence. This suppresses the orbital fat signal and reduces chemical shift artifact.

Thirty-seven adults with a recent or past episode of optic neuritis underwent MR imaging. Eight patients had other features of clinically probable or definite MS. The most frequent clinical features of optic neuritis were pain, an afferent pupillary defect, a central scotoma, and impaired color vision (table). Focal lesions were found on MR imaging in 37 of 44 symptomatic optic nerves and in 6 of 30 asymptomatic nerves. No additional lesions were found using a gadolinium-enhanced $T_1$-weighted sequence. Lesions were found in 25 of 31 nerves involved by a recent attack, and in 12 of 13 patients in whom the attack occurred more than 3 months previously.

Magnetic resonance imaging demonstrates optic nerve lesions in most patients with optic neuritis. However, visual evoked potential recording is the preferred study. Abnormal MR signals probably result from edema in acute lesions of the central nervous system and from gliosis in chronic lesions.

▶ Here is yet another expensive test to add to other evaluations, such as visually evoked responses, that are superfluous to the diagnosis and management of optic neuritis. Optic neuritis remains a clinical diagnosis, established by a thorough neuro-ophthalmic history and examination. No disease controls such as ischemic, infiltrative, or compressive optic neuropathies were examined. Presently, use of the STIR sequence should be considered investigational.—R.C. Sergott, M.D.

| Optic Neuritis: Clinical Features in 44 Nerves | |
| --- | --- |
| Orbital pain | 37/42 (88%) |
| Afferent pupillary defect | 31/35 (89%) |
| Impaired color vision | 27/38 (71%) |
| (Ishihara) | |
| Visual field (confrontation) | |
| Central scotoma | 28/38 (74%) |
| Other abnormality | 5/38 (13%) |
| Normal | 5/38 (13%) |
| Worst VA < 6/60 | 23/39 (59%) |
| Disk swelling | 13/31 (42%) |
| Good recovery (VA ≥ 6/9) | 38/44 (86%) |
| Fast recovery (26) | |
| Slow recovery (10) | |
| Poor recovery (VA < 6/9) | 6/44 (14%) |

(Courtesy of Miller DH, Newton MR, van der Poel JC, et al: *Neurology* 38:175–179, February 1988.)

### Optic Neuropathy in Chronic Lymphocytic Leukemia

Currie JN, Lessell S, Lessell IM, Weiss JS, Albert DM, Benson EM (Natl Eye Inst, Bethesda, Md; Mental Health Research Inst, Victoria, Australia; Massachusetts Eye and Ear Infirmary, Boston; Lahey Clinic, Burlington, Mass; Monash Univ, Victoria)

*Arch Ophthalmol* 106:654–660, May 1988                4–9

Ophthalmologic and neurologic involvement is infrequent in chronic lymphocytic leukemia (CLL) and usually occurs late in the course of disease. In 3 patients, progressive visual loss from optic nerve infiltration was an early clinical finding of CLL. All 3 patients had progressive optic atrophy with loss of acuity and the visual field, preceded in 1 case by transient visual obscurations and disk edema.

In 1 patient with diffuse optic nerve enlargement on computed tomography, histopathologic examination showed an infiltrate of small, generally mature lymphocytes in the major vessels within the nerve and smaller vessels within the septas. Phenotype study showed that these cells were of monoclonal B-cell origin. The cerebrospinal fluid (CSF) in this patient contained 34 white cells per cubic millimeter, 94% of them lymphocytes. Similar CSF findigs were obtained in all 3 cases.

Optic neuropathy was one of the earliest clinical manifestations of CLL in these patients, although 2 of the 3 had had leukemia for longer than 10 years. Worsening of the CLL accompanied the appearance of optic neuropathy. Once visual loss begins, rapid and aggressive treatment is necessary. All 3 patients had significant improvement in acuity and expansion of the visual field after optic nerve irradiation, although each had residual optic atrophy.

▶ The clinical rule that "a neuro-ophthalmic problem in a patient with cancer is caused by the cancer until proven otherwise" is again validated. Radiation therapy produced visual improvement. Therefore, this entity is an important cause of treatable visual loss. Compared with previous reports, these patients are unique, because the optic neuropathy occurred "early" in the course of their disease.—R.C. Sergott, M.D.

### Progressive and Recurrent Nonarteritic Anterior Ischemic Optic Neuropathy

Borchert M, Lessell S (Massachusetts Eye and Ear Infirmary, Boston)

*Am J Ophthalmol* 106:443–449, October 1988                4–10

Nonarteritic anterior ischemic optic neuropathy usually results in precipitous visual loss. The visual defect is either maximal when first noted or evolves over hours to days; rarely does progression occur over weeks. Ten patients were described with nonarteritic anterior ischemic optic neuropathy in whom the visual deficit progressed over a number of weeks or who had recurrence of disease in the same eye.

In 5 patients the visual deficits progressed over 1 month or more; 4 patients had recurrence of disease in the same eye after a long interval; and 1 had bilateral progression and recurrence. Temporal artery biopsy tissue showed no evidence of arteritis in 6 patients. The other 4 in whom biopsy was not performed, had normal erythrocyte sedimentation rates. Although it has been assumed that the ischemia and functional loss stop abruptly, these findings suggested that they may not.

These 10 patients with nonarteritic anterior ischemic optic neuropathy had recurrence of disease in the same eye or progression over intervals ranging from weeks to months.

The incidence of recurrence and progression of anterior ischemic optic neuropathy in the same eye might be higher than is generally appreciated.

▶ This study confirms previous observations (Boghen DR, Glaser JS: *Brain* 98:689, 1975) that in some patients nonarteritic ischemic optic neuropathy worsens over several weeks. This is important to remember so that patients are not subjected to excessive neuroradiologic testing. Perhaps nonarteritic ischemic optic neuropathy is not entirely "ischemic," as has been assumed for many years.—R.C. Sergott, M.D.

---

## The Management of Optic Nerve Sheath Meningiomas

Kennerdell JS, Maroon JC, Malton M, Warren FA (Allegheny Gen Hosp, Pittsburgh; Charlotte Mem Hosp, Charlotte, NC; New York Univ, New York)
*Am J Ophthalmol* 106:450–457, October 1988                    4–11

---

The orbital optic nerve sheath meningioma is difficult to treat because of its location and unpredictable biologic activity. The results of treatment were reviewed in 38 patients with 39 affected eyes after follow-up of at least 3 years.

Eighteen eyes were simply observed because they had minimal functional deficit or were blind. Nine patients had an initial visual acuity of 20/50 or worse, and 7 of these patients had severe, long-standing, partial or complete visual loss. At initial examination, only 2 had visual acuity of better than 20/100; both declined radiotherapy. One patient in this group had a visual acuity of 20/50 despite a severe superior visual field defect. Visual acuity subsequently declined to counting fingers at 6 ft, with minimal change in visual field. Six patients with optic nerve sheath meningiomas confined to the orbit received radiotherapy, about 5,500 rad in 28–32 treatments. All patients had progressive visual field loss or decreasing visual acuity before therapy and improved visual acuity and visual fields afterward. Improved visual function was maintained for at least 30–84 months. None of the patients had reduced visual function or tumor growth on computed tomography. The tumor did not shrink markedly after radiation. The only complication was 1 transiently dry eye. In 6 other patients surgery was performed initially in an attempt to remove optic nerve sheath meningiomas but was abandoned.

In this series all 6 patients with optic nerve sheath meningiomas treated with radiotherapy alone had improved visual acuity or visual fields for

3–7 years. Tissue diagnosis does not appear to be necessary before proceeding with external beam irradiation, provided that computed tomographic and magnetic resonance imaging findings are characteristic of optic nerve meningioma. At present, there is no optimal way to treat optic nerve sheath meningiomas.

▶ This study presents promising data for the use of radiation therapy for optic nerve sheath meningiomas, a previously untreatable cause of blindness. However, larger series of patients are still needed to establish this modality as the treatment of choice. Clinicians should remember that the dose of radiation delivered is potentially damaging to the intraocular contents and could also induce radiation necrosis of the optic chiasm and contralateral optic nerve. Therefore, this treatment should be administered only by radiation therapists with extensive experience using radiation in and around the orbit.—R.C. Sergott, M.D.

---

**Modified Optic Nerve Sheath Decompression Provides Long-Term Visual Improvement for Pseudotumor Cerebri**
Sergott RC, Savino PJ, Bosley TM (Wills Eye Hosp, Philadelphia)
*Arch Ophthalmol* 106:1384–1390, October 1988                4–12

---

Twenty-three patients with chronic papilledema and pseudotumor cerebri underwent a modified optic nerve sheath decompression procedure. Rather than removing a single section of optic nerve meninges, at least 3 longitudinal incisions were made in the sheath, and arachnoidal adhesions were lysed with a tenotomy hook within the subdural space.

All but 2 patients had improved visual function after initial decompression. The mean follow-up was 21.5 months. In the 2 patients who failed to improve initially a single meningeal window was made, and improvement followed reoperation with the modified method. Twelve of 21 patients with bilateral visual loss had improved vision bilaterally after unilateral operation; 6 patients required bilateral surgery. Disk pallor did not predict a poor operative outcome. Six responsive patients failed to recover vision after lumboperitoneal shunting.

Long-term visual improvement can be expected after this modified optic nerve decompression operation. The need for systemic steroid therapy is much reduced. The unoperated-on eye also often improves. The procedure can succeed where lumboperitoneal shunting has failed.

---

**Optic Nerve Sheath Decompression: How Does it Work? Has Its Time Come?**
Keltner JL (Sacramento, Calif)
*Arch Ophthalmol* 106:1365–1369, October 1988                4–13

---

Pseudotumor cerebri causes serious visual loss in up to one fourth of affected patients and lesser impairment in as many as half of them. Optic nerve sheath decompression appears to be an effective means of relieving visual impairment in these patients. Both the older literature and current work support the view that optic nerve sheath fenestration locally decompresses the optic nerve by filtration. Variable decompression of the 3-compartment subarachnoid system takes place. The extent of decompression depends on resistance from trabeculations in the subarachnoid space of the optic nerve sheath in both the optic canal and the orbit.

Previously, lumboperitoneal shunting has been used to treat pseudotumor cerebri. Shunt revision has been necessary in a varying proportion of patients. Optic nerve sheath decompression may be preferable when visual function declines despite maximum medical treatment, including oral diuretics and possibly a trial of oral prednisone. Either the medial or the lateral route may be effective. The complication rate is low. Headaches frequently improve after the decompression procedure. Surgery probably should be done soon after medical treatment fails, because normal vision may not return if chronic atropic papilledema develops.

---

**Results of Optic Nerve Sheath Fenestration for Pseudotumor Cerebri: The Lateral Orbitotomy Approach**

Corbett JJ, Nerad JA, Tse DT, Anderson RL (Univ of Iowa; Univ of Utah; Bascom Palmer Eye Inst, Miami)
*Arch Ophthalmol* 106:1391–1397, October 1988                4–14

---

Twenty-eight patients with pseudotumor cerebri underwent 40 optic nerve sheath fenestration procedures to relieve visual loss or to preserve vision. Twelve patients had bilateral operations. A change of at least 2 lines in acuity was considered significant.

Acuity was improved or unchanged after optic nerve sheath fenestration in 85% of eyes. Acuity improved in 12 eyes and remained the same in 22, but it declined in 6 eyes after surgery. Only 3 to 8 eyes with preoperative acuity of 20/200 or worse improved. Visual fields improved in 21 eyes and remained the same in 10. Two eyes with preserved acuity had field loss. Nine of 17 patients with bilateral disk swelling had improvement in papilledema in the unoperated eye. One patient had retrobulbar hemorrhage postoperatively. There were no infections. Headaches were relieved in 11 of 17 patients.

Optic nerve sheath fenestration is indicated in patients with progressive loss of acuity or visual field or with pseudotumor cerebri. If severe visual loss is present vision may not improve, but may be preserved by fenestration. Surgery also is indicated for the appearance of new field defects and for an increasing afferent pupillary defect.

► Optic nerve sheath decompression surgery has had a controversial past, with many advocates and detractors. Now, multiple centers with several surgeons performing basically the same procedure, nerve sheath decompression, report encouraging and similar results in pseudotumor cerebri. Although the mechanism(s) by which the procedure resolves severe papilledema remains unknown, it now is clear that the operation succeeds when maximal medical therapy or lumboperitoneal shunts fails. Because the procedure can produce blindness, it should not be performed unless loss of visual field and acuity is documented.—R.C. Sergott, M.D.

**Treatment of Carotid-Cavernous Sinus Fistulas Using a Detachable Balloon Catheter Through the Superior Ophthalmic Vein**
Hanneken AM, Miller NR, Debrun GM, Nauta HJW (Wilmer Ophthalmological Inst, Baltimore; Johns Hopkins Med Insts)
*Arch Ophthalmol* 107:87–92, January 1989                    4–15

Four patients with carotid-cavernous sinus fistulas not amenable to endoarterial balloon occlusion or embolization were treated successfully by advancing a detachable balloon catheter through the ipsilateral superior ophthalmic vein. Three patients had a spontaneous fistula and the fourth had a traumatic fistula. The balloon was passed into the cavernous sinus under angiographic control, inflated to close the fistula, and detached. There were no deaths and morbidity did not occur. Symptoms and signs resolved completely in all cases.

The endoarterial route is not always feasible, and a direct approach to the cavernous sinus carries significant risks. Transvenous passage via the inferior petrosal sinus may not be possible. The present patients had orbital dissection to identify an anterior segment of the superior ophthalmic vein and free it from surrounding orbital tissues using the operating microscope.

The team includes an orbital surgeon, neurosurgeon, and interventional neuroradiologist. Possible complications include puncture of the superior ophthalmic vein with severe bleeding and loss of vision, infection, and damage to anterior orbital structures.

**Paradoxic Pupillary Phenomena: A Review of Patients With Pupillary Constriction to Darkness**
Frank JW, Kushner BJ, France TD (Univ of Wisconsin)
*Arch Ophthalmol* 106:1564–1566, November 1988                    4–16

Pupillary constriction in darkness may occur in either retinal disease or optic nerve disease. It is described in patients with congenital stationary night blindness, congenital achromatopsia, bilateral optic neuritis, or dominant optic atrophy. In a series of 29 patients, the initial response to darkness was pupillary constriction. Direct and consensual responses to light and the near response were normal.

In 25 of 29 patients the paradoxic response was associated with abnormality of the optic nerve or retina, or with nystagmus. Seven patients had congenital stationary night blindness or achromatopsia, and 6 had anomalies of optic nerve development. Six patients had congenital nystagmus and 6 had various retinal disorders. Four patients had strabismus and amblyopia but no apparent retinal or optic nerve disease. There was no personal or family history of nyctalopia.

The finding of paradoxic pupillary constriction in darkness in patients without retinal or optic nerve abnormalities questions its value as a localizing sign for such disease.

## Tonic Upgaze in Infancy: A Report of Three Cases

Ahn JC, Hoyt WF, Hoyt CS (Univ of California, San Francisco)
*Arch Ophthalmol* 107:57–58, January 1989                    4–17

Transient supranuclear disorders of gaze occur in healthy infants. Three infants were seen who had episodic conjugate tonic upgaze in the first months of life without seizures or downgaze palsy. The episodes became more brief and less frequent with advancing age, occurring most notably during times of illness or fatigue.

Tonic upgaze deviation in these infants may be analogous to the transient tonic downward deviation seen in otherwise healthy infants. Upward deviation lasts longer than downward deviation. Upward deviation is also described as part of seizure activity, in postencephalitic parkinsonism, in children with bilateral central visual loss caused by retinal disease when the inferior field is relatively preserved, and in states of coma. It also occurs in brain stem disease producing downgaze palsy.

## Blepharospasm: A Review of 264 Patients

Grandas F, Elston J, Quinn N, Marsden CD (King's Coll Hosp Med School and Moorfields Eye Hosp, London)
*J Neurol Neurosurg Psychiatry* 51:767–772, June 1988          4–18

Blepharospasm now is considered a neurologic disorder. Data were reviewed on 264 patients having a mean age at onset of 56 years. Females predominated in this series. Dystonia elsewhere was present in 78% of patients, most often in the cranial-cervical region. About 10% of patients had a family history of blepharospasm or dystonia elsewhere. Ocular lesions preceded the onset of blepharospasm in 12% of the patients. In one fifth there was a unilateral onset, with spread to the other eye after a mean of 2 years. Factors such as bright lights, television viewing, and reading increased spasms in many instances, whereas sleep and relaxation frequently led to improvement. Nineteen patients had blepharospasm secondary to Parkinson's disease.

Responses to drugs were inconsistent, although one fifth of the patients given anticholinergics improved initially (Table 1). All but 2 of 29 bilateral facial nerve avulsion operations led to improvement, but recurrence was the rule. Botulinum toxin injections produced significant improvement in a large majority of patients (Table 2). Benefit lasted for a mean

TABLE 1.—Drug Treatment of Blepharospasm

| Drug | No. Patients Treated | No. Patients With Benefit | % |
|---|---|---|---|
| Anticholinergics | 96 | 20 | 20.8 |
| Levodopa | 34 | 7 | 20.6 |
| Lisuride | 14 | 4 | 28.6 |
| Bromocriptine | 7 | 1 | 14.3 |
| Tetrabenazine | 52 | 3 | 5.7 |
| Haloperidol | 28 | 4 | 14.2 |
| Pimozide | 36 | 2 | 5.5 |
| Chloropromazine | 7 | 1 | 14.3 |
| Antidepressants | 25 | 3 | 12 |
| Benzodiazepines | 38 | 3 | 7.8 |
| Propranolol | 14 | 1 | 7 |
| Lithium | 6 | 1 | 16.7 |

The effects of drug treatment were assessed by retrospective review of the case records. All patients were treated with maximum tolerated doses of the individual drugs. Benefit was defined as the restoration of some useful vision.

(Courtesy of Grandas F, Elston J, Quinn N, et al: *J Neurol Neurosurg Psychiatry* 51:767–772, June 1988.)

of 9 weeks. Persistent disabling problems occurred in 15% of the patients.

A genetic predisposition is possible in a minority of patients with blepharospasm. Evaluation of drug treatment is complicated by spontaneous remissions, reported in 11% of the present series. Botulinum toxin injection is an effective approach, but most patients require treatment about 5 times a year.

▶ This is a very large study of blepharospasm, a fairly common problem and one quite frustrating to ophthalmologists. The study reconfirms the success of botulinum toxin in alleviating symptoms in a large majority of patients. This is an excellent overall review of blepharospasm that gives good data concerning clinical features, symptoms, drug treatment, and surgery for this disease. In the end, botulinum toxin seems to work best, although repeated injections are usually necessary.—P.R. Laibson, M.D.

TABLE 2.—Effects of Botulinum Toxin Injections on Vision in 151 Patients With Blepharospasm

| Degree of Improvement | No Patients (%) |
|---|---|
| 75%–100% | 55 (36.4) |
| 50%–75% | 39 (25.8) |
| 25%–50% | 24 (15.9) |
| Less than 25% | 11 (7.3) |
| Unknown (follow-up too short) | 22 (14.6) |

*The degree of improvement was assessed by prospective estimation of the percentage of the waking day spent functional blind, before and after the injection of botulinum toxin injections.

(Courtesy of Grandas F, Elston J, Quinn N, et al: *J Neurol Neurosurg Psychiatry* 51:767–772, June 1988.)

# 5  Oculoplastics

## YAG Contact and Argon Lasers in Ophthalmic Plastic Surgery

Joseph C. Flanagan, M.D., F.A.C.S.
*Cornea Department, Wills Eye Hospital, Philadelphia, Pennsylvania*

An invaluable tool that has been added to the armamentarium of the ophthalmic plastic surgeon is the yttrium/aluminum/garnet (YAG) contact laser, which is used in conjunction with the argon laser. Most lasers presently used by ophthalmologists are the Q-switched or mode-locked, ultra-pulsed type that are capable of delivering extremely short bursts of high-peak energies to precise target areas. The argon laser has its principal energy output at a wavelength of 4,880–5,145 Å. This is in the green-blue range of the visible spectrum. The energy transfer involves electrical energy being transformed into light energy within the laser, and this is transformed into thermal energy, which causes protein coagulation in the target tissues. Selective absorption of the green-blue light by the hemoglobin of erythrocytes creates a thermal effect that results in vessel obliteration. Because of this, the argon laser is extremely useful in treating vascular malformations and tumors. Other lesions that have been treated successfully with the argon laser include port-wine hemangiomas, superficial varicose veins, capillary and cavernous hemangiomas, superficial telangiectasis, pyogenic granulomas, seborrheic keratoses, senile angiomas, rosacea, and tattoos.

Unfortunately, the argon laser is not as effective in the treatment of patients with very dark complexions because the green-blue light is absorbed by melanin. This selective absorption provides a wide margin of safety, however, with regard to damage to surrounding tissues in patients with light complexions. Vascular lesions can be treated with low-power settings, with little destruction of surrounding tissues and scar tissue formation. Because greater power is required to treat dark areas or lesions (e.g., tattoos, seborrheic keratoses, or nevi), the risk of tissue damage and scarring is higher.

The YAG contact laser functions in a different manner in that the laser energy is focused and concentrated at the tip of a synthetic sapphire probe. The probe is used as a surgical scalpel to cut, vaporize, or coagulate tissue and affords the same tactile sensation as conventional scalpels. Because cutting, vaporization, and coagulation occur at the visible tip of the probe, surgical techniques do not have to be modified in any way from those already used by the surgeon. The main advantage of the YAG contact laser is that blood loss can be minimized. This is most useful when performing operations that can be associated with significant blood loss such as dacryocystorhinostomy, excision of vascular lesions, or debulking of orbital tumors. It also helps to reduce operating time and morbidity among patients with coagulation disorders and among those who must use anticoagulant medications.

The interaction of light from a laser with the target tissue depends on the output power, the area or spot size of the beam, the laser wavelength, and the absorption characteristics of the tissue. The power density from the YAG contact laser can be varied by changing the configuration of the probe tip or the power output. With proper adjustment of these variables, the desired effect of cutting, coagulation, or vaporization can be achieved. Because the YAG laser can affect tissue to a depth of 3–5 mm, it is particularly effective in maintaining hemostasis, even when active bleeding is encountered.

## Argon Laser

Pretreatment consultation with the patient and family members is extremely important. This should include thorough discussion of the goals and risks of treatment, as well as possible alternative therapies. Cosmetic considerations may be of primary concern and should be reviewed in detail. In addition, the physician must understand the patient's expectations, so that any misconceptions can be dispelled before treatment has been initiated. Pretreatment and posttreatment photographs are essential for patient counseling and documenting the final results. Informed consent must be obtained as in any other surgical procedure.

Most argon laser procedures are performed in the office or other outpatient setting. Local anesthesia, consisting of the subcutaneous injection of 2% xylocaine without epinephrine, is used for most patients. Regional blocks and topical anesthetic paste or sprays are not satisfactory. General anesthesia may be necessary for children, or when several different areas of the body are treated during a single session. For relatively large lesions (e.g., a nevus flammeus), a test area approximately 2 cm in diameter can be treated and observed for a period of 4 months. A decision to proceed with treatment of the entire lesion can then be made with greater certainty that the final results will be satisfactory.

Patients are instructed to wear no makeup on the day of the procedure. The area to be treated is prepped with sterile saline before the local anesthetic solution is injected. Everyone present in the treatment area, including the patient, must wear protective goggles while the laser is used. When treating eyelid lesions, the contralateral eye is covered with a patch saturated with saline solution and the ipsilateral eye is protected with a scleral shell. Some investigators believe that application of ice compresses immediately before treatment may enhance the effects of laser therapy. However, conclusive evidence as to the efficacy of chilling the skin has not been forthcoming.

For vascular lesions the average power setting is 1 W. Damage to surrounding tissues is minimal, as is scarring, with powers this low. Pigmented lesions (e.g., seborrheic keratoses, nevi, and tattoos) require higher settings, in the range of 3 W. Consequently, the risk of damage to surrounding tissues and scarring is greater. When treating lesions of the eyelids and orbital area, an intermittent technique is usually used. Pulses are applied in a linear fashion so that the areas of blanching from each pulse approximate one another but do not overlap. The pulse duration is generally 0.2 second and the interval between pulses is 0.5 – 1.0 second. In treatment of large lesions a continuous pulse may be delivered. The beam is passed across the skin at a rate that allows blanching to be observed. With the intermittent method, the power setting and duration of the pulse can be adjusted to achieve an optimal level of blanching. The power setting and speed at which the beam is passed can be adjusted when the continuous method is used. The end point of blanching occurs with vascular lesions and signifies vessel obliteration caused by thermal protein coagulation. For other lesions the end point is not as clearly defined. This can lead to excessive treatment with damage to surrounding tissues. Unfortunately, some damage to normal tissue may be unavoidable when removing tattoos because treatment must extend into the dermis to achieve satisfactory destruction of the tattoo.

Some postoperative discomfort is to be expected from the second-degree burn, which is a component of laser treatment. This can usually be relieved with nonprescription analgesics, but occasionally more effective medications are required. Most authors believe that ice compresses, applied four times per day, are helpful in limiting swelling in the periorbital area, a site more prone to swelling than most other areas of the body. A topical antibiotic ointment is used in the morning and at bedtime during the early postoperative period. Although a nonadherent dressing (e.g., Telfa) can be applied, we usually do not dress lesions in the periorbital area. The patient is instructed to wash the treated area gently twice daily with sterile saline solution. The first postoperative visit is at 1 week, or sooner if the patient observes any untoward effects.

## YAG Contact Laser

Preoperative evaluation and postoperative care are the same as when conventional surgical techniques are used. The advantages and limitations of the laser should be discussed with the patient, and informed consent must be obtained. During the procedure, protective goggles must be worn by everyone present, including the patient. For operations that involve the eyelids or periorbital area, the patient's eyes can be protected with patches or scleral shells, as previously described when using the argon laser. Intraoperatively, the power setting should be adjusted or the probe tips changed to achieve the desired effect of cutting, coagulation, or vaporization.

Because the use of the YAG contact laser possibly may delay wound healing, we now remove sutures a few days later than usual. However, wound appearances more than 2 or 3 weeks postoperatively have not been observed to differ from those of patients who have not had laser therapy.

*Suggested Reading*

Bartlett JA, Ridins KH, Salkeld LJ: Management of hemangiomas of the head and neck in children. *J Otolaryngol* 17:11 – 20, 1988.
Dicken CH: Argon laser treatment of port wine stains. *Mayo Clin Proc* 60:115 – 117, 1985.

Federman JL: Contact laser surgery with potential application in ophthalmology. *Contemp Ophthalmic Forum* 4:97–100, 1986.
Gilchrest BA: Laser therapy for selected cutaneous vascular lesions in pediatric population: A review. *Pediatrics* 82:652–662, 1988.
Gladstone GJ, Beckman H: Argon laser treatment of an eyelid margin capillary hemangioma. *Ophthalmic Surg* 14:944–946, 1983.
L'Esperance F Jr: *Ophthalmic Lasers.* St Louis, CV Mosby, 1983.
Peyman GA, Katoh N, Tawakol M, et al: Contact Nd:YAG laser for use in oculoplastic surgery. *Jpn J Ophthalmol* 31:635–645, 1987.
Silver L: Argon laser photocoagulation of port wine stain hemangiomas. *Lasers Surg Med* 6:24–28, 52–55, 1986.

## Radiotherapy of Periocular Basal Cell Carcinomas: Recurrence Rates and Treatment With Special Attention to the Medial Canthus

Rodriguez-Sains RS, Robins P, Smith B, Bosniak SL (Manhattan Eye, Ear and Throat Hosp; New York Univ, New York)
*Br J Ophthalmol* 72:134–138, 1988                    5–1

Basal cell carcinomas of the medial canthal region can spread deeply into the orbit and sinuses and eventually require exenteration for cure. Many recurrent lesions at this site have previously been irradiated, and the recurrent tumors appear to be unusually aggressive and destructive.

Among 631 consecutive biopsy-proved basal cell carcinomas of the eyelids were 55 recurrent tumors that were primarily irradiated. Most of the patients were treated definitively by Mohs' surgery, conventional surgery, or both. Of 127 primary untreated tumors in the medial canthal region, 6 recurred. The recurrence rate in 116 previously treated medial canthal lesions was 9.5%. Seven of 42 irradiated medial canthal tumors recurred.

The best chance of totally eradicating a tumor is at initial presentation if an aggressive approach is taken. Excision of basal cell carcinoma of the eyelid monitored by frozen section control should be undertaken or Mohs' surgery should be carried out. Radiotherapy may remain useful in some cases. However, medial canthal lesions have a higher recurrence rate and are more likely to invade the orbit; they should be managed in such a way that tissue is sampled to ensure adequate treatment.

► Radiation therapy should be reserved for elderly patients because of the possibility of radiation complications developing many years later. Aggressive surgical excision with pathologic monitoring is preferred, particularly in medial canthal lesions; however, radiation therapy may be used under extenuating circumstances.—J.C. Flanagan, M.D.

## Metastatic Squamous Cell Carcinoma of the Conjunctiva

Tabbara KF, Kersten R, Daouk N, Blodi FC (King Saud Univ, Riyadh; King Khaled Eye Specialist Hosp, Riyadh Saudi Arabia)
*Ophthalmology* 95:318–321, March 1988                    5–2

Regional metastasis from conjunctival squamous cell carcinoma is rare, as is distant metastasis. However, 10 Saudi Arabian patients aged 45–75 years with this cancer had regional or distant metastasis. The initial metastatic sites included the parotid and submandibular glands, preauricular and cervical lymph nodes, lungs, and bone (table, p 88). Six patients had previously had excision of conjunctival squamous cell carcinoma. Orbital extension was noted in 8 patients.

Squamous cell cancer of the conjunctiva appears to be more aggressive in Saudi Arabia than elsewhere, probably because of delayed treatment. Regional metastasis does not necessarily carry a poor prognosis. Increased exposure to ultraviolet light may help to explain the increased incidence in thermal/tropical regions. Primary total resection is the best management. Close follow-up allows early detection of recurrent disease. If node involvement is detected early enough, radical neck dissection may provide a cure before distant metastasis develops. In addition, ultraviolet-blocking lenses are used prophylactically.

▶ Patient delay is the principal cause of metastases in squamous cell carcinoma of the conjunctiva. Prophylaxis with the use of ultraviolet-light-blocking lenses should be stressed, as well as early detection and aggressive primary treatment.—J.C. Flanagan, M.D.

## Mechanism of Orbital Blow-Out Fracture: Experimental Study by Three-Dimensional Eye Model

Fujino T, Sato TB (Keio Univ, Tokyo)
*Orbit* 6:237–246, 1987

5–3

Converse and Smith proposed that orbital blow-out fracture results from a sudden rise in intraorbital pressure caused by traumatic force applied to the orbital soft tissues. However, some findings cannot be explained in this way. A 2-dimensional eye model was designed resembling a cut section of the human skull from the midpart of the infraorbital margin to the optic canal. A 3-dimensional model study was done to confirm the findings in the 2-dimensional model. The orbital walls were studied alone, with the orbital contents, and also with the eyeball present.

When various sites received an impact, the force applied to the eyeball alone did not increase the infraorbital hydraulic pressure sufficiently to cause an orbital floor fracture. When the infraorbital margin was struck, however, the orbital floor was displaced laterally and finally fractured by bending stress. Even at this point the increased hydraulic pressure did not account for orbital floor fracture.

These experiments suggest that orbital floor fracture is secondary to bending stress rather than to an increase in infraorbital pressure itself.

▶ A new mechanism of orbital blow-out fracture has been described. It has been alluded to elsewhere in the literature, and this article explains the patho-

Squamous Cell Carcinoma of the Conjunctiva in 10 Patients

| Case No. | Age/Sex | Site of Initial Lesion | Intraocular/ Orbital Involvement | Site of Metastasis | Previous Surgery | Management |
|---|---|---|---|---|---|---|
| 1 | 61/M | OS (total)* | +/+ | Parotid | Excision of conjunctival lesion (1X) | Exenteration Parotidectomy Radiation |
| 2 | 55/M | OD (nasal limbus) | +/− | Parotid | Excision of conjunctival lesion (2X) | Enucleation Radiation Chemotherapy |
| 3 | 65/F | OD (inferonasal limbal area) | −/+ | Preauricular lymph node | Excision of conjunctival squamous cell carcinoma (2X) | Exenteration Parotidectomy |
| 4 | 60/F | OD (temporal and inferior limbus) | +/+ | Preauricular lymph node Cervical lymph node | None | Exenteration Parotidectomy Radical neck dissection |
| 5 | 75/F | OD (total)* | +/+ | Bone Lungs Preauricular lymph nodes | Excision of conjunctival lesion (2X) | Palliative radiation Open reduction of pathologic fracture (patient died 8 mos later) |
| 6 | 54/M | OD (inferonasal) | +/− | Preauricular and cervical lymph nodes Parotid | Excision of conjunctival lesion (1X) | Radical neck dissection Radiation therapy |
| 7 | 66/M | OD (total) | +/+ | Preauricular lymph node Parotid | None | Exenteration Parotidectomy Radiation |
| 8 | 75/M | OD (inferonasal limbal area/fornix) | −/+ | Submandibular cervical lymph nodes | Enucleation | Radiation Radical neck dissection Exenteration |
| 9 | 50/F | OS (temporal limbus/ inferior fornix) | −/+ | Submandibular and preauricular lymph nodes | None | Radical neck dissection Radiation |
| 10 | 45/M | OS (nasal limbus) | +/+ | Cervical and submandibular lymph nodes | None | Exenteration Radical neck dissection Radiation |

OS, left eye; OD, right eye.
*Total destruction of ocular surface by tumor.
(Courtesy of Tabbara KF, Kerten R, Daouk N, et al: *Ophthalmology* 95:318–321, March 1988.)

physiology of an orbital floor fracture on clinical and experimental grounds.—J.C. Flanagan, M.D.

## Lid Retraction Following Blow-Out Fracture of the Orbit

Conway ST (Tufts Univ)
*Ophthalmic Surg* 19:279–281, April 1988                    5–4

Enophthalmos with pseudoptosis is an established complication of blow-out fracture of the orbit. Retraction of the upper lid is a paradoxic response that has been described only twice previously. A third such patient was seen who had a different response to treatment.

Putterman and Urist believed that lid retraction in 2 patients was secondary to overaction of Mueller's muscle. Both patients were cured by a Meuller's muscle excision. This procedure was ineffective in the third patient, suggesting that the disorder resulted from traction on the connective tissue sheath of the levator palpebrae through its interconnections with the connective tissue system of the other extraocular muscles. The levator connective tissue system may be pulled posteriorly by downward fraction forces from the connective tissue of the inferior rectus muscle, transmitted at the apex. Recession of the levator aponeurosis significantly reduced lid retraction in the third patient after Mueller's muscle resection failed.

▶ Lid retraction also could be explained by the superior rectus muscle and levator muscle pulling against a fibrotic or entrapped inferior rectus. This is one of the mechanisms that causes retraction of an upper eyelid in thyroid ophthalmopathy and may be the mechanism in this case. In this instance, recession of the levator aponeurosis should significantly reduce eyelid retraction, as was the case in this presentation.—J.C. Flanagan, M.D.

## Ocular Injuries in Boxing

Smith DJ (Wills Eye Hosp, Philadelphia)
*Int Ophthalmol Clin* 28:242–245, Fall 1988                    5–5

Despite much discussion about the harmfulness of boxing, no large, properly conducted study of the medical effects of boxing has been carried out. Data were examined on 118 boxers and dilated ophthalmoscopy was performed in 68 of them.

Overall, 21% of the boxers had marked ocular damage. Cataract formation was most prevalent, and the most common type of opacity was posterior subcapsular cataract. Nineteen percent of the boxers examined had vitreoretinal injury. Five had retinal tears, and 5 had old vitreous hemorrhage. The boxers with ocular damage had not had many more fights than the others, but total exposure time was impossible to determine.

Cataract formation in a boxer may be secondary to equatorial expansion. Retinal injuries apparently reflect both contrecoup damage and equatorial expansion. Contrecoup forces also may lead to cyst formation in the central retina. Ocular injuries occur frequently in boxers. All boxers should wear a protective helmet and eyeguard while sparring.

▶ The incidence of ocular injuries among boxers is high, and a dilated fundus examination, slit-lamp examination, and intraocular pressure check are essential in the routine examination of anyone involved in this sport. The same evaluation and precautions hold true in the management of any patient who sustains blunt trauma to the orbital area.—J.C. Flanagan, M.D.

---

**Dysthyroid Optic Neuropathy: The Crowded Orbital Apex Syndrome**
Neigel JM, Rootman J, Belkin RI, Nugent RA, Drance SM, Beattie CW, Spinelli JA (Univ of British Columbia, Vancouver)
*Ophthalmology* 95:1515–1521, November 1988                    5–6

---

Optic neuropathy is a serious complication of Graves' disease that requires immediate treatment. The role of apical orbital crowding was studied in 58 patients who had dysthyroid optic neuropathy in 95 eyes. The control group included 60 patients (119 eyes) with thyroid orbitopathy but not optic neuropathy; all 60 had computed tomography studies during the previous 2 years.

Patients with optic neuropathy were seen later than those with usual orbitopathy, with a later onset of thyroid eye disease. They were more likely to be male and diabetic. Deteriorating color vision was a frequent presenting feature. Asymmetric extraocular muscle restriction and vertical tropias were characteristic of patients with neuropathy. Computed tomography confirmed that crowding at the orbital apex was associated with optic neuropathy. Proptosis was substantially more marked in orbits with neuropathy.

Marked proptosis, palpable lacrimal glands, substantial restriction of extraocular muscles, and vertical tropia should suggest optic neuropathy in patients with thyroid eye disease. In addition, there is a greater increase in intraocular pressure on upgaze. Computed tomography shows apical crowding as well as enlarged muscles and anteriorly displaced lacrimal glands. The diameter of the superior ophthalmic vein is increased. Visual evoked potential recording is the most sensitive means of detecting early optic neuropathy.

▶ To detect optic neuropathy as early as possible, it is extremely important to evaluate the color vision when examining patients with thyroid ophthalmopathy. If there is evidence of optic nerve damage, medical, surgical, or radiation decompression of the orbit should be considered. When vision is threatened, surgical decompression is best performed through a Caldwell-Luc approach, so that the posterior orbital floor and the medial wall of the orbit may be decompressed to alleviate pressure at the posterior aspect of the orbit.—J.C. Flanagan, M.D.

## Surgical Approaches to Diseases of the Orbital Apex
Leone CR Jr, Wissinger JP (Univ of Texas, San Antonio)
*Ophthalmology* 95:391–397, March 1988                                    5–7

Orbital masses deep in the apex may be difficult to expose and are best approached transcranially. The standard frontal craniotomy may be used, as well as a modified supraorbital transcranial approach. The latter involves removal of the superior rim and roof of the orbit, exposing all but the orbital floor. The chief indication is a mass deep in the orbital apex that would be difficult or impossible to expose adequately by conventional orbitotomy. The frontal sinus is exenterated and packed with fat from the thigh before coverage with pericranium. In the standard craniotomy, a polypropylene screen is used to restore the orbital roof.

A transcranial approach to disease in the orbital apex can be used in patients who otherwise would be candidates for a direct orbital approach. A controlled break is made across the anterior roof in place of an unpredictable break posteriorly that might damage structures within the apex or lacerate the dura. No infections or extrusions have occurred to date, and there has been no serious morbidity. The procedure is done extradurally, lowering the complication rate. However, ophthalmic morbidity is often unavoidable.

▶ Exposure and biopsy of small lesions at the orbital apex may be extremely difficult without causing serious problems with vision and extraocular motility. All too often there are reports that an orbitotomy has been performed, but the biopsy results were negative for pathologic material. This combined ophthalmologic and neurosurgical approach should be strongly considered to expose small lesions at the orbital apex surgically.—J.C. Flanagan, M.D.

## Orbital Myositis Involving the Oblique Muscles: An Echographic Study
Wan WL, Cano MR, Green RL (Univ of Southern California; Doheny Eye Inst, Los Angeles)
*Ophthalmology* 95:1522–1528, November 1988                              5–8

Idiopathic orbital myositis is a frequent nonspecific form of orbital inflammation that can involve 1 or more extraocular muscles but usually not the oblique muscles. Computed tomography shows diffuse enlargement of the affected muscles with contrast enhancement, and echography shows homogeneous low-reflective enlargement of the muscles and tendons.

Seven of 30 patients with idiopathic orbital myositis had involvement of the inferior or superior oblique muscle. On initial examination 2 patients had bilateral involvement of the oblique muscles. Other muscles were involved in all cases but 1. Each involved muscle showed the typical homogeneous low-reflective echo of myositis, with variable degrees of thickening. The episclera was often thickened as well.

Orbital myositis usually responds to systemic steroid therapy, but the restriction of gaze may persist. Recurrences are fairly frequent after an initial response. Irradiation or immunosuppressive drug therapy may be indicated in refractory cases.

▶ When orbital myositis is diagnosed by computed tomography findings or echography, treatment in the form of high-dose systemic steroids is usually instituted. If there is not a significant relatively rapid response or if there is recurrence, biopsy of the involved area should be considered to rule out other causes of muscle enlargement or simulated muscle enlargement such as metastatic carcinoma or other malignancies. If orbital myositis is diagnosed pathologically, reinstitution of high-dose systemic steroids, radiation, or immunosuppressant drugs should be planned.—J.C. Flanagan, M.D.

---

**Chronic Hematic Cyst of the Orbit: Role of Magnetic Resonance Imaging in Diagnosis**
Kersten RC, Kersten JL, Bloom HR, Kulwin DR (Univ of Cincinnati; Fort Hamilton-Hughes Mem Hosp, Hamilton, Oh)
*Ophthalmology* 95:1549–1553, November 1988                                              5–9

---

Chronic hematic cysts are uncommon lesions that usually are not suspected before operation. The cysts enlarge progressively, leading to expansion or erosion of the orbital bones, and may appear on computed tomography scans as a malignant orbital process (Fig 5–1). On magnetic resonance (MR) imaging a high signal is seen on T1- and T2-weighted images, with the appearance being essentially pathognomonic of hematic cyst.

These cysts consist of old blood and blood breakdown products with granulomatous response and a surrounding fibrous pseudocapsule. Probably, blunt trauma leads to orbital bleeding that is incompletely absorbed. The clinical picture is nonspecific; painless, progressive, unilateral proptosis usually occurs over months to years. Chronic accumulation of blood characteristically produces high signal intensity on MR images.

When malignancy of the lacrimal glands is ruled out, the blood products, granulomatous response and fibrous pseudocapsule may be removed. The lesion has not recurred after evacuation.

▶ Scanning with computed tomography (CT) is still the single most useful imaging technique for orbital disease. However, neural tumors and uncommon problems, such as a hematic cyst, may have pathonomonic appearances on MR imaging. Before exploring an orbit surgically, the CT scan should be supple-

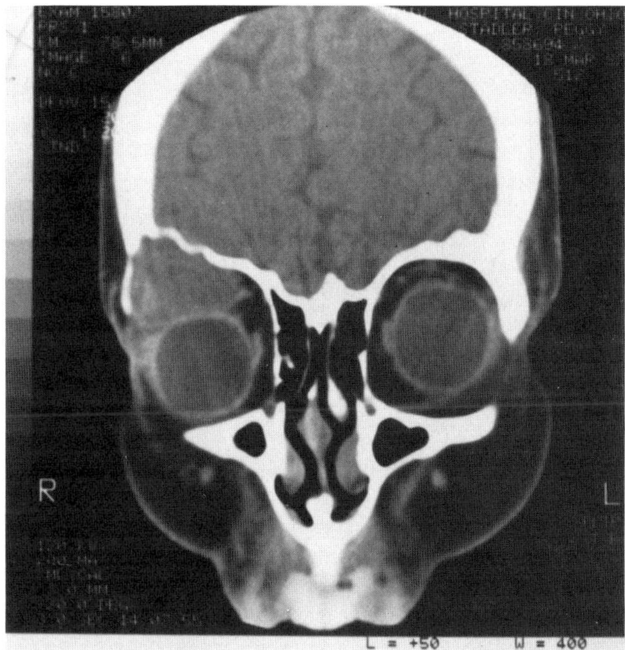

Fig 5–1.—Woman aged 38 years. Coronal CT scan demonstrating superior right orbital mass with erosion and expansion of lateral aspect of right orbital roof. (Courtesy of Kersten RC, Kersten JL, Bloom HR, et al: *Ophthalmology* 95:1549–1553, November 1988.)

mented with an MR scan if there is any question about the findings.—J.C. Flanagan, M.D.

---

## Technique for Incisional Biopsy of a Lacrimal Gland Mass When the Diagnosis of Benign Mixed Tumor Cannot Be Excluded Clinically

Tse DT, Folberg R (Univ of Iowa)
*Ophthalmic Surg* 19:321–324, May 1988                                        5–10

---

In some patients with a lacrimal gland mass it is necessary to obtain an incisional biopsy to exclude a benign mixed tumor. A technique was developed with the goal of preventing tumor spillage in the event tumor has to be removed. The incision site is covered with several drops of butyl–2–cyanoacrylate. The specimen is submitted for frozen section study. If a benign mixed tumor is present, the entire gland may be removed (table), with the cyanoacrylate bond protecting the lacrimal gland contents from contaminating the orbit. If an inflammatory pseudotumor is found (Fig 5–2), there is a permanent seal over the lacrimal gland incision site.

Incisional biopsy is not indicated if the history and radiologic findings clearly support a diagnosis of benign mixed tumor. In addition, frozen

Algorithm for Incisional Biopsy of Lacrimal Gland Mass With Frozen Section

I.  If the frozen section diagnosis is inflammatory pseudotumor:
   A.  The surgeon closes the lateral orbitotomy wound in the standard fashion.
      1.  The butyl-2-cyanoacrylate forms a permanent seal over the lacrimal gland incision site.
   B.  If the permanent sections confirm the diagnosis of pseudotumor, no further surgery is necessary.
   C.  If the permanent sections reveal benign mixed tumor, the lateral orbitotomy site is opened and the lacrimal gland with adjacent periorbita is removed en bloc.
      1.  The butyl-2-cyanoacrylate seal may be reinforced with an additional application of tissue adhesive.
      2.  Butyl-2-cyanoacrylate has the tensile strength to withstand subsequent manipulation without dislodging from the incision site.
II.  If the frozen section diagnosis is equivocal:
   A.  Close the lateral orbitotomy site in standard fashion.
   B.  If permanent sections reveal inflammatory pseudotumor, no additional surgery is necessary.
   C.  If permanent sections reveal benign mixed tumor, proceed as in step I-C.
III.  If the frozen section diagnosis indicates unequivocal benign mixed tumor:
   A.  Reinforce the lacrimal gland incision site with additional butyl-2-cyanoacrylate.
   B.  Remove the entire lacrimal gland with adjacent periorbita.

(Courtesy of Tse DT, Folberg R: *Ophthalmic Surg* 19:321–324, May 1988.)

sections should not be used routinely to diagnose lacrimal gland tumors. Tissue adhesive should be used only if there is a possibility of incising into a benign mixed tumor. Close cooperation with an ophthalmic pathologist is important.

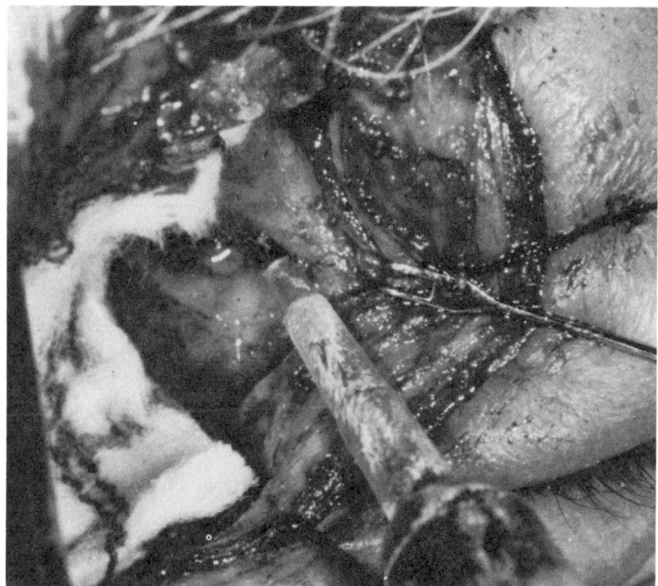

Fig 5–2.—Photograph taken after frozen section indicating inflammatory pseudotumor. Neurosurgical cottonoids have been removed from 1 edge of the gland in preparation for closure of the lateral orbitotomy wound. The tip of the tissue adhesive applicator is in the position used earlier to apply the butyl-2-cyanoacrylate. (Courtesy of Tse DT, Folberg R: *Ophthalmic Surg* 19:321–324, May 1988.)

▶ This is an excellent procedure to follow in patients with a lacrimal gland mass that does not fit into the algorithm used by many orbital surgeons. It gives the surgeon the opportunity to biopsy a lacrimal gland mass without spilling cells into surrounding tissues. If a routine open biopsy is performed on a benign mixed tumor of the lacrimal gland, the patient may be subjected to repeated episodes of orbital surgery because of local recurrences of the tumor. The pathologist sectioning the tissue should be familiar with lacrimal gland pathology.—J.C. Flanagan, M.D.

## Hemifacial Spasm Due to Intracranial Tumor: An International Survey of Botulinum Toxin Investigators

Sprik C, Wirtschafter JD (Univ of Minnesota)
*Ophthalmology* 95:1042–1045, August 1988                    5–11

Hemifacial spasm usually is benign, but rarely it is caused by an intracranial mass lesion. Because botulinum toxin investigators frequently see patients with hemifacial spasm and no other neurologic deficits, a survey was carried out in 1,676 patients so affected.

Nine tumors were reported, for an incidence of 0.5%; most were in women older than 50 years. However, computed tomography (CT) or magnetic resonance imaging (MRI) was performed in only about half of the patients. No single tumor type predominated.

Computed tomography with intravenous contrast medium is an adequate means of examining patients with hemifacial spasm for intracranial tumor, but MRI eliminates much of the bone artifact. If 1 in 200 patients with hemifacial spasm has a tumor and an MRI or CT study costs $500, detection of just 1 lesion would cost $100,000.

▶ Any woman older than 50 years of age with hemifacial spasm of short duration should have an MRI scan to rule out any intracranial disease. If there are other symptoms, however, such as hearing loss, complete neurologic evaluation should be performed. The incidence of serious neurologic problems in these patients is low; however, such disease should be ruled out before injection of botulinum toxin.—J.C. Flanagan, M.D.

---

**Nasolacrimal Drainage System Obstruction After Orbital Decompression**
Seiff SR, Shorr N (Univ of California, San Francisco and Los Angeles)
*Am J Ophthalmol* 106:204–209, August 1988                              5–12

---

Data on 63 patients with dysthyroid ophthalmopathy were reviewed after 123 orbital decompression procedures. The most frequent indications were exposure keratopathy and cosmesis. Eighty-four transantral ethmoidal decompressions and 33 transconjunctival orbital decompressions were carried out.

All patients with compressive optic neuropathy had definite improvement after transantral decompression. Sixteen percent of transantral ethmoidal decompressions were followed by epiphora, which began 11–18 months postoperatively. All of these patients had obstruction distal to the common internal punctum. Complete obstruction was present in 7 patients. All 10 dacryocystorhinostomies led to symptomatic relief.

The delayed onset of epiphora after transantral orbital decompression suggests progressive scarring of the nasolacrimal drainage system, leading to obstruction. Damage to adjacent tissues probably causes scarring to extend into this area. Transantral decompression is not necessarily more risky than other means of orbital decompression, inasmuch as it is usually performed in patients with severe dysthyroid ophthalmopathy.

▶ In orbital decompression transantral decompression is the most effective method of dealing with optic neuropathy secondary to thyroid ophthalmopathy, and even though nasolacrimal duct obstruction may occur, the transantral approach should be considered in these patients. When orbital decompression is being performed for cosmetic reasons, a superior approach through the internal cul-de-sac is effective and is not associated with nasolacrimal duct obstruction.—J.C. Flanagan, M.D.

**Dacryocystography After Paranasal Sinus Surgery**
Hunink MGM, de Vries-Knoppert WAEJ, Balm AJM, Luth WJ (Academic Hosp of the Free Univ, Amsterdam)
*Br J Radiol* 61:362–365, May 1988                    5–13

Lacrimal dissection is performed during lateral rhinotomy or transantral ethmoidectomy to remove paranasal tumors. The effects of lacrimal duct dissection on lacrimal drainage were assessed in 19 patients who had recently undergone these operations. One patient had bilateral surgery. Both dye tests and dacryocystography were used. In 10 patients the contralateral side was evaluated.

Nearly all patients had an abnormal lacrimal system at the operative site and 5 had obstruction. Only 1 patient not given radiotherapy had obstruction, and this patient had undergone 2 additional operations for recurrence. In 4 of 10 patients given postoperative radiotherapy canalicular obstruction developed.

The lacrimal system is injured during paranasal sinus surgery, but in most patients obstruction of the drainage system does not develop. The nasolacrimal duct often is shortened and the lacrimal sac displaced, but without apparent physiologic sequelae. Irradiated patients might have prophylactic intubation of the lacrimal system at the time of paranasal sinus surgery.

▶ Lacrimal gland obstruction is not uncommon in any type of sinus or nasal surgery. It may follow cosmetic rhinoplasty, especially if an osteotomy is used to narrow the nasal bridge. Transnasal or anterior ethmoidal sinus surgery commonly cause dacryostenosis because of the proximity of the ethmoid air cells to the lacrimal fossa.—J.C. Flanagan, M.D.

---

**Allergic Lacrimal Obstruction**
Wojno TH (Emory Clinic, Atlanta)
*Am J Ophthalmol* 106:48–52, July 1988                    5–14

It is generally presumed that epiphora, or lacrimal hypersecretion, is a response to stimulation by the offending allergen in allergic conjunctivitis. However, intermittent epiphora may occur in response to temporary obstruction at the level of the lacrimal sac or canaliculus, initiated by rubbing the periocular tissues.

Five patients with a documented history of atopic disease and a long-standing history of intermittent epiphora reported that the tearing was accompanied by itching, particularly in the medial canthi. All 5 patients underwent initial lacrimal testing when symptom free. Each patient was then asked to return for reexamination when symptoms suggestive of allergic conjunctivitis reappeared, but with the specific instruction not to rub the eyes, even momentarily, on the day of examination. While in the office under observation the patient was allowed to rub the pruritic ocular tissues of the right medial canthus for only 30 seconds. All 5 patients experienced the onset of epiphora within 5 minutes, and lacrimal testing was then repeated.

When asymptomatic the patients had no evidence of lacrimal obstruction. However, at retesting only the symptomatic, rubbed eye showed both overflow tearing, as confirmed by the basic secretion tear test, and remarkable prolongation in the dye disappearance test. The primary dye test yielded positive results bilaterally in all 5 patients when asymptomatic, but negative results only in the eye that had been rubbed for 30 seconds. The nonrubbed nasolacrimal system remained patent even though the eye was equally pruritic. The test results were suggestive of unilateral lacrimal obstruction. The epiphora cleared within 4 hours if rubbing was not repeated.

Three patients given cromolyn sodium eyedrops reported complete relief of epiphora and symptoms of ocular irritation. In patients with ocular allergy, rubbing the pruritic medial canthal tissues could promote further contact of allergen with the mucosa of the lacrimal sac and canaliculi. This could increase mast cell degranulation and release of vasoactive amines. The combination of eye rubbing and ocular anaphylaxis might thus potentiate the effect that each alone would have. Cromolyn sodium, a mast cell stabilizer and blocker of the allergic response, relieves the urge to rub the eyes and consequently breaks the cycle that leads to edema in the lacrimal system.

▶ This mechanism should be considered in the workup in patients complaining of epiphora in the presence of a patent nasolacrimal system. A therapeutic trial of cromolyn sodium eyedrops may be helpful in patients with functional nasolacrimal duct obstruction patent to irrigation.—J.C. Flanagan, M.D.

---

**Histopathological Findings in Blepharopigmentation (Eyelid Tattoo)**
Hurwitz JJ, Brownstein S, Mishkin SK (Univ of Toronto; McGill Univ)
*Can J Ophthalmol* 23:267–269, October 1988                    5–15

It has become popular to tattoo eyelids for cosmetic reasons by implanting iron oxide pigment into the lid at the level of the lash follicles. Three patients were treated by excising the affected area after intervals of 1 hour, 5 days, and 18 months. Pigment remained as free epidermal and dermal granules in the early specimens (Fig 5–3). At 18 months most residual pigment was present in dermal macrophages and in the endomysial connective tissue of the superficial orbicularis oculi. There was no significant damage to treated tissues.

There is no evidence that eyelid tattooing has significant adverse local effects. No more than minimal muscle damage or inflammation was seen after 18 months, the longest interval between tattooing and pathologic assessment.

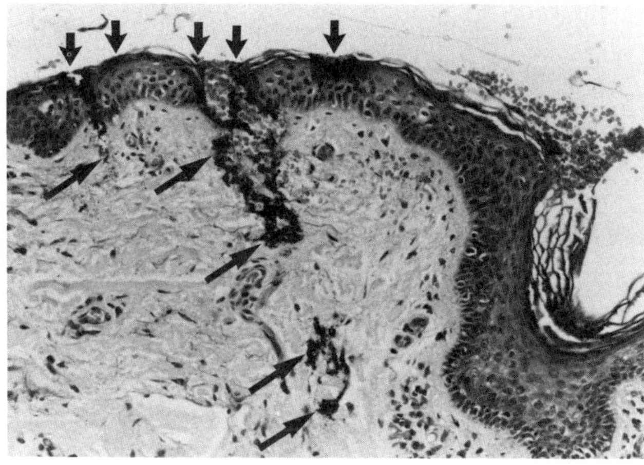

**Fig 5–3.**—Eyelid specimen obtained 5 days after tattooing showing focal disruption of epidermis, which contains clusters of pigment granules *(short arrows)* that extend into adjacent dermis *(long arrows)* and stain positive for iron Prussian blue; ×200, reduced by approximately 50%. (Courtesy of Hurwitz JJ, Brownstein S, Mishkin SK: *Can J Ophthalmol* 23:267–269, October 1988.)

► To date, no significant changes have been reported as a result of blepharopigmentation with iron oxide pigment. One important consideration is this: Can it be reversed, or can the iron oxide pigment be removed if the patient no longer desires this tattoo of the eyelid? Surgical excision is difficult and leaves scars, and laser treatment has not been helpful to date. Therefore, the patient should be informed that this is a nonreversible process at this time.—J.C. Flanagan, M.D.

## The Surgical Treatment of Blepharoptosis in Oculomotor Nerve Palsy

Malone TJ, Nerad JA (Univ of Iowa)
*Am J Ophthalmol* 105:57–64, January 1988                5–16

Data were reviewed on 170 patients with congenital and acquired oculomotor nerve palsy diagnosed between 1961 and 1986. Congenital palsy was present in 16% of patients, and 70% of these patients were amblyopic. Of 20 patients who had surgery for blepharoptosis, 15 had congenital and 5 had acquired oculomotor nerve palsy.

The state of levator muscle function was the chief factor in the choice of surgical procedure. Four patients without measurable levator function underwent sling operations. The other patients had levator muscle resection or advancement of the aponeurosis. One patient who refused a frontalis sling procedure had a Whitnall sling operation. Four patients with aberrant regeneration had persistent synkinetic lid movements despite successful repair of blepharoptosis. Only 1 patient was reoperated on. Six patients had corneal complications; all of them were undercorrected.

In acquired blepharoptosis surgery is done only after the neurologic deficit has stabilized. Exposure keratitis is a significant complication of any operation for blepharoptosis. The risk of corneal complications can be lowered by minimizing postoperative lagophthalmos. Eyebrow suspension and supermaximal levator muscle resection carry a greater risk of lagophthalmos than do levator muscle aponeurosis advancements with good levator muscle function. Lid elevation to a purely cosmetic level is not wise in a patient with poor levator muscle function.

▶ If there is a significant vertical or horizontal ocular deviation, it should be corrected as much as possible before ptosis surgery. If the lid is elevated in the presence of a large extraocular muscle deviation, corneal exposure is more likely to occur and cosmesis will be less than optimum. Undercorrection may be beneficial because of a poor to absent Bell's phenomenon.—J.C. Flanagan, M.D.

---

**Silicone Gel Sheet Tie-Over for Skin Graft on the Eyelid Following Release of Scar Contracture**
Sawada Y (Hirosaki Univ, Japan)
*Br J Plast Surg* 41:325–326, 1988                                               5–17

---

A tie-over dressing is useful in fixing a graft to the recipient bed, but the grafted skin cannot be inspected directly and it may be difficult to detect hematoma at an early stage. The use of a translucent silicone gel sheet solves this problem.

*Technique.*—After suturing the graft in place, elastic translucent silicone gel sheet is cut to the shape of the graft and placed on it. Several layers may be used if desired. Sutures are tied with the ends left long for easy removal if a hematoma is seen. The graft is sandwiched between the silicone sheet and tarsus and fixed closely to the recipient bed. Tarsorrhaphy and a light dressing with absorbable material are recommended. If a hematoma develops, the sutures are untied and removed, the hematoma expressed, and the silicone sheet reapplied.

No infection has occurred with this technique. The method may be used on small flat defects anywhere on the body surface. It is especially applicable to eyelid grafts after releasing scar contracture, because the grafted skin is firmly fixed between the tarsus and the silicone sheet.

▶ Some type of pressure dressing is essential over a free full-thickness skin graft for 5 days to allow capillary invasion into the bed of the graft. This sheet is one type that is available to ensure equal pressure over the graft, and has the advantage of allowing visualization of the grafted area. Surgeons are often tempted to remove such dressings early to inspect the state of the graft; this is not recommended. It replaces the necessity of a pressure dressing over the entire eye area and allows the patient to use the eye if a tarsorrhaphy has not been performed as part of the integral procedure.—J.C. Flanagan, M.D.

## Blepharochalasis

Bergin DJ, McCord CD, Berger T, Friedberg H, Waterhouse W (Letterman Army Med Ctr, Presidio of San Francisco; Emory Univ)
*Br J Ophthalmol* 72:863–867, 1988                    5–18

Blepharochalasis is an uncommon disorder in which young patients have recurrent episodes of eyelid edema that are not associated with pain or erythema. Eventually, the lid skin becomes redundant, atrophic, and discolored. Blepharoptosis occurs despite excellent levator function. A hypertrophic form with fat herniation also is recognized.

Four female patients with blepharochalasis of the atrophic type were

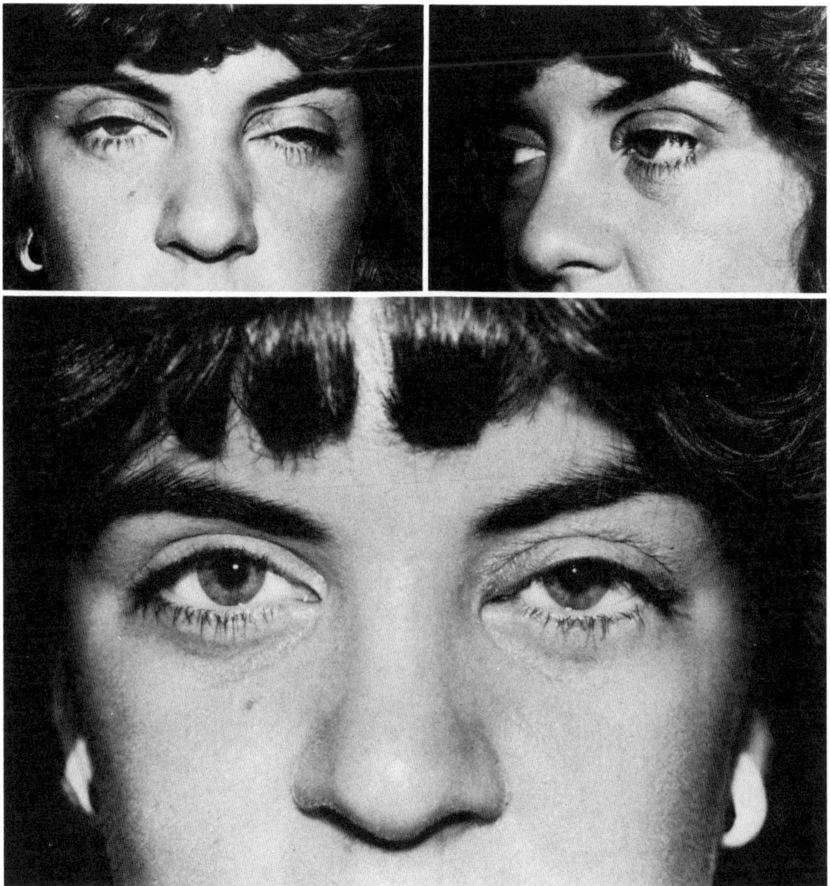

Fig 5–4 (top).—Woman aged 20 years. **Left,** photograph shows ptosis, redundant atrophic eyelid skin, and high superior tarsal lid crease. **Right,** lateral view shows nasal fat pad atrophy, pseudoepicanthal fold, and rounded lateral canthal angle.

Fig 5–5 (bottom).—Same patient as in **Fig 5–4.** Photograph obtained 6 months after 4-lid blepharoplasty, external levator aponeurosis tuck, dermis fat graft, and lateral canthoplasty.

(Courtesy of Bergin DJ, McCord CD, Berger T, et al: *Br J Ophthalmol* 72:863–867, 1988.)

managed by an external levator aponeurosis tuck, blepharoplasty, lateral canthoplasty, and dermal fat grafting. All had increased vascularity and decreased dermal elastic fibers, even in the papillary dermis. An external approach to the levator aponeurosis tuck provides good exposure and may be combined with an upper lid blepharoplasty through the same incision. When the skin edges are fixed to the edge of the levator aponeurosis, symmetric lid creases are achieved (Figs 5–4 and 5–5). More dermis than fat should be used; an additional 30% overcorrection usually is optimal. A lower lid blepharoplasty is done in conjunction with lateral canthoplasty if the lower lid skin is redundant. Lateral canthotomy, inferior cantholysis, and lateral horizontal shortening of the lid are done if required.

▶ Blepharochalasis is common and causes both cosmetic and functional problems in otherwise young and healthy patients. Both cosmetic and functional factors can usually be corrected with external levator plication and blepharoplasty surgery. For the occasional surgeon, the dermis fat graft may in certain cases be a formidable procedure, and I am sure the patient would be just as happy with the results of external levator plication and blepharoplasty. Because of the variable absorbtion of the dermis fat graft, titration is difficult, even for the most experienced surgeon.—J.C. Flanagan, M.D.

---

**Botulinum Toxin A-Induced Protective Ptosis in Corneal Disease**
Kirkness CM, Adams GGW, Dilly PN, Lee JP (Moorfields Eye Hosp and St George's Hosp Med School, London)
*Ophthalmology* 95:473–480, April 1988                                    5–19

---

Corneal epithelial defects that fail to heal cause much ocular morbidity, and the resultant scarring or infection may lead to loss of vision. The usual methods of encouraging reepithelialization entail risk to the eye or to structures of the lid margin. Botulinum toxin protective ptosis (BTPP) was evaluated in 25 patients who otherwise would have been considered for surgical tarsorrhaphy. Botulinum toxin A produces temporary flaccid ptosis when injected into the levator palpebrae superioris muscle. Toxin was injected just below the central part of the superior orbital rim.

Twenty-one patients had indolent corneal ulceration, and 4 with neuroparalytic keratitis were treated prophylactically. Ninety percent of the indolent ulcers healed completely. Complete ptosis was produced in three fourths of the eyes within an average of 3½ days and lasted for an average of 16 days. Levator function recovered completely within an average of 8½ weeks. Superior rectus underaction recovered completely within 6 weeks. Impression cytologic studies showed much improvement in patients with ulceration. None lost vision as a result of the procedure.

Botulinum toxin protective ptosis is an effective means of covering the cornea in patients with resistant ulcers and of aiding reparative processes. The eye is readily examined, and medications instilled. Botulinum toxin protective ptosis may be indicated for treating refractory corneal ulcers and to protect eyes exposed by neurologic dysfunction.

▶ Ptosis may be a temporary complication when botulinum toxin A is injected into the eyelid area in patients with severe primary essential blepharospasm. The ptosis generally clears up in approximately 2 weeks and is mild in nature. In the treatment of corneal ulcers, the use of eyelid sutures may be just as effective without risking permanent ptosis or other complication (e.g., diplopia) that could occur with injection of botulinum toxin in the ocular area.—J.C. Flanagan, M.D.

# 6  Oncology

## The Multicenter, Prospective, Randomized Clinical Trial

JAMES J. AUGSBURGER, M.D.
*Wills Eye Hospital, Philadelphia, Pennsylvania*

The most widely discussed topic in ocular oncology during the past several years has been that of multicenter prospective randomized clinical trials of management options for patients with choroidal and ciliary body melanoma. In the following paragraphs, I would like to present my impressions of both the pros and cons of such an investigation.

### The Basis of Randomized Clinical Trials

The randomized clinical trial is a planned experiment on human subjects in which the primary purpose is to determine the relative merits of alternative treatments. The essential elements of a clinical trial include (1) control patients who either receive no treatment, conventional treatment, or a placebo; (2) random assignment of patients to the treatments to be tested; (3) no clear evidence before the trial favoring one treatment over the other in terms of the outcomes in question; and (4) a firm ethical basis for the research. Randomization in a clinical trial effectively ensures that the personal judgment and prejudices of the investigators do not influence the allocation of patients to the treatment modalities under study. Consequently, any difference between patients in a clinical trial will result from either random chance or the true relative effectiveness of the treatments and not to susceptibility bias.

The general ethical justification for randomized clinical trials is the judgment that, in certain conditions for which two or more treatments exist without clear evidence showing which is best in terms of the outcome or outcomes of interest, it is legitimate for the physician to advise his or her patients to enroll in a well-designed clinical experiment that can answer that question, provided that the patient has been fully informed about the current state of knowledge of the relative effectiveness and complications of the treatments, because of the overriding need of society for progress in disease control (1).

Randomized clinical trials are most appropriately applied to studies of relatively common conditions that are associated with one or more important clinical end points that occur in a substantial number of affected patients within a reasonably short period of time (2,3). In ophthalmology, conditions that appear to fall within these guidelines include diabetic retinopathy and macular degeneration. Both of these conditions have been and currently are under investigation in randomized clinical trials.

The benefits that can be derived from randomized clinical trials include

(1) benefits to the participants, and (2) benefits to potential future patients. The principal direct benefits to participants in well-designed and fastidiously performed randomized clinical trials include a consistently high standard of care rendered to all those enrolled and limitation of the risk of receiving the worse treatment to 50%. Exceptional clinical trials (e.g., the Diabetic Retinopathy Study) taht randomize treatment to a paired organ that tends to be affected relatively symmetrically actually provide every enrolled patient a 100% chance that he or she will receive the better treatment. The true principal value of a patient's participation in a randomized clinical trial, however, appears to be the knowledge that his or her participation will benefit future affected patients, and society in general, by enabling physicians to determine which treatment is better, what the magnitude of that treatment differential is, and what the relative complications experienced by patients managed by competing treatments are.

During the past 15 years randomized clinical trials have become thoroughly established, universally admired, sometimes revered, and frequently criticized (4). The universal admiration for well-designed randomized clinical trials arises from the many obvious benefits they have brought to medical research and clinical practice; the list of therapeutic interventions for various conditions shown to be ineffectual by randomized clinical trials is far too extensive to be cited here. Some enthusiasts of randomized clinical trials appear to regard these studies with a reverence resembling religious devotion (4) (a phenomenon I occasionally refer to as "the religion of clinical trials"). These enthusiasts tend to want any new treatment to be evaluated by a randomized clinical trial, starting with the first patient. Furthermore, they commonly urge physicians and patients to accept no evidence about therapeutic efficacy unless it comes from randomized clinical trials.

## Criticisms of Randomized Clinical Trials

Criticism of randomized clinical trials has come from multiple sources and for many reasons, including conflicts in the design and analysis of the trials, unhappiness about controversies in which the trials have raised more questions than they answered, complaints about their costliness and potential stifling of creativity, and concerns about every aspect of their ethics, ranging from recruitment to long-term follow-up of treated patients. Even the most antagonistic critics of randomized clinical trials today, however, usually focus on specific problems, rigidities, or other inadequacies of trial design, analysis, or interpretation and do not recommend abandonment of clinical trials or a return to the pretrial era. A full discussion of the criticisms of randomized clinical trials is beyond the scope of this commentary. The reader is referred to Feinstein (4) (pp 691–709) for a detailed discussion of the common criticisms.

The principal criticism of most randomized clinical trials is their ethical basis. Feinstein has described the fundamental conflict about the ethics of clinical trials in terms of *societal* versus *samaritan* viewpoints (4). In the societal viewpoint, clinicians are obligated to find and demonstrate worthwhile agents of therapy. In the samaritan viewpoint, clinicians are obligated to do their best for individual patients. Both of these viewpoints can be justified but the two frequently cannot be reconciled. Both viewpoints are completely ethical, but they collide regularly during decisions about whether, when, and how to do a randomized clinical trial. In the samaritan viewpoint, randomization itself is often an unacceptable method of choosing therapy because it removes clinical judgment from choices tailored to the nuances of a patient's personal needs. Because these individualized samaritan judgments have led to the many past delusions about therapeutic merits, however, randomization is welcomed from the societal viewpoint as a prime mechanism for avoiding the delusions. Although proponents of the samaritan approach may claim that certain treatments are too well established to warrant randomized clinical trials, adherents to the societal viewpoint can cite a long list of well-established treatments that were eventually shown, often with randomized trials, to be useless or even harmful.

The societal-samaritan conflict also occurs when informed consent is sought from patients solicited to enter a trial (4). Because randomized trials are almost always conducted with the suspicion that one treatment is superior to another and because sample sizes are calculated on the basis of that suspicion, advocates of the samaritan viewpoint believe that clinicians seeking a patient's informed consent are not being completely truthful in stating that the trial is intended merely to see whether a difference exists between the two treatments. The societal viewpoint, however, can ethically justify a statement that the trial is intended to provide convincing evidence of a difference and to detect unsuspected complications.

Another conflict between the societal and samaritan viewpoints arises when there is doubtful feasibility of a proposed clinical trial. If the condition or disorder of interest is uncommon, the outcome event or events of interest in that disorder are infrequent during a relatively short time interval; the difference between the outcome event rates of patients treated by the alternative method is expected to be small based on previous nonrandomized but statistically adjusted comparison studies. The feasibility of enrolling a sufficient numer of patients and following them to the pertinent end point events, so that a clinically meaningful and statistically valid result will be obtained, may be extremely low. Adherents to the societal viewpoint may believe that it is worthwhile to perform such a study despite its low feasibility, because failure to do so will leave clinicians and their patients in perpetual uncertainty as to which treatment is truly better. Proponents of the samaritan viewpoint may conclude that the low probability of recruiting and following a sufficient number of participants to provide a meaningful and statistically significant result in a randomized clinical trial is a misuse of patients, which presents an ethical contraindication to their participation (5).

Another common criticism of randomized clinical trials is the validity of generalization of results (4). Because of the eligibility and exclusionary criteria of a randomized clinical trial, the results of a particular clinical trial are scientifically valid only for patients comparable in all aspects to those in the trial treated by the methods employed in the trial. Such results cannot be extrapolated with validity to patients different from those studied in the trial or to patients managed by different therapeutic options.

### Application of Randomized Clinical Trial Methodology to the Study of Posterior Uveal Melanomas: The Collaborative Ocular Melanoma Study

As I mentioned in my introductory comments, it has been suggested that a randomized clinical trial should be considered whenever there is a *balance* between physicians who believe that a particular form of treatment for a specific condition or disorder should be used and those who are uncertain or believe that the harm of that treatment may outweigh its benefit. This may well be the case for choroidal and ciliary body melanoma (6). There is certainly no consensus at this time regarding the "best" treatment for patients with this tumor. At one extreme are a few zealous ophthalmologists who fervently *believe* enucleation to be the only treatment that should be offered to patients with posterior uveal melanoma and who emphatically proclaim that any other intervention worsens the patient's chance of survival (7). At the other extreme are some "ophthalmic oncologists" who appear to believe that "conservative" (potentially eye-preserving) therapeutic interventions are preferable to enucleation in most patients with posterior uveal melanoma (8). Most ophthalmologists are uncertain and confused and wish to have the issue resolved. From this perspective, there seems no question that randomized clinical trials should be considered as a means of assessing the true relative effectiveness of competing treatments for posterior uveal melanoma.

In response to this collective uncertainty about the relative effectiveness of enucleation and various "conservative" treatments for patients with posterior uveal melanoma, a number of proponents of randomized clinical trials designed what is now known as the Collaborative Ocular Melanoma Study (COMS) (9). This study, which is supported by the National Eye Institute (NEI), has as its cornerstone a randomized clinical trial of enucleation versus iodine-125 plaque radiotherapy for patients with an intermediate size choroidal melanoma. The COMS also includes a clinical trial of enucleation alone versus enucleation after oculo-orbital photon irradiation for patients with a large choroidal or ciliary body melanoma and a nonrandomized prospective study of patients with a small posterior uveal melanoma. The basic design of the COMS has been reported in the ophthalmic literature (9), and virtually all ophthalmologists in the United States and Canada have also received direct mailings to announce the study. The COMS steering group has recruited multiple clinicians to take part in this study, and the participating centers have been enrolling patients since 1987.

### My Objections to the COMS

I have three major objections to the COMS: (1) the disregard for current evidence in its design, (2) the apparently intentional exclusion of many of the foremost "ocular oncologists" in the United States, and (3) the limited value of any result that may be obtained.

DISREGARD FOR CURRENT EVIDENCE

The COMS was designed by enthusiasts for randomized clinical trials who had very little collective personal experience with potentially eye-preserving ("conservative") management methods for patients with posterior uveal melanoma. These individuals minimized the value of evidence available at that time from several nonrandomized but statistically adjusted comparison studies showing no appreciable benefit of enucleation over ocular tumor radiotherapy in terms of melanoma-specific mortality rates.[8, 10–12] By doing so, the designers of the COMS were able to justify specifying a substantially larger experimental treatment differential than is likely to be observed. This justification in turn led them to estimate a required sample size substantially lower than the number of patients actually likely to be needed for a clinically meaningful and statistically significant result. Using this dubious estimate, however, they were able to convince the NEI that they could recruit a sufficient number of patients to proceed with their experiment.

My viewpoint on this issue is distinctly in line with the samaritan philosophy (4). If the true differential effect of enucleation and plaque or charged particle radiotherapy on survival in patients with a medium-size choroidal melanoma is as small as suggested by all of the nonrandomized but statistically adjusted comparative studies reported to date, then it is highly unlikely that the COMS will be able to recruit, treat, and follow enough patients with such a tumor for a long enough time to show with a scientifically acceptable degree of certainty (e.g., alpha $\leq$ 0.1, beta $\leq$ 0.05) that a clinically important difference in favor of enucleation does not exist. Stated alternatively, the most likely result of the COMS enucleation versus iodine-125 plaque radiotherapy trial of medium-size choroidal melanomas is an inadequate result (13), one that leaves unanswered the question, "Do I take the eye out or leave it in?" I believe it is unethical to ask patients to participate in the COMS enucleation versus iodine-125 plaque radiotherapy trial because it has only a small chance of detecting a treatment differential unless it is substantially larger than that predicted by virtually all of the nonrandomized but statistically adjusted comparative survival studies currently available (5).

EXCLUSION OF MANY OF THE FOREMOST "OCULAR ONCOLOGISTS" IN THE UNITED STATES

The COMS manual of procedures demands that participating clinical investigators agree in writing to attempt to enroll all eligible patients with a posterior uveal melanoma in the appropriate component COMS randomized clinical trial. This requirement effectively excludes many of the foremost "ocular oncologists" in this country (Gragoudas, Seddon, and coworkers at the Massachusetts Eye & Ear Infirmary, Boston; Char and coworkers, University of California, San Francisco; Ellsworth, Coleman, and coworkers at the Cornell University—New York Hospital Medical

Center, New York City; and Shields, myself, and our coworkers at Wills Eye Hospital, Philadelphia) who routinely employ treatment methods other than enucleation and iodine-125 plaque radiotherapy in many patients with a medium-size choroidal melanoma. Although many individuals participating in the COMS are well-known clinicians and researchers, very few have substantial experience with plaque radiotherapy of posterior uveal melanomas and virtually none has a clinical practice devoted almost exclusively to the diagnosis and management of ophthalmic tumors. A randomized clinical trial that does not enjoy the active support of a majority of the foremost experts in the field of investigation must certainly be viewed by casual observers with some degree of skepticism as well as amusement.

THE LIMITED VALUE OF ANY RESULT THAT MAY BE OBTAINED

Despite their many splendid and admirable accomplishments, randomized clinical trials have substantial limitations that arise from the limited spectrum of scientific challenges to which the trials can be successfully applied (4). Although invaluable for appraising many issues in therapy, randomized clinical trials cannot be used effectively for answering all questions that occur in patient care. Not even the most complete scientific description of the relative impact of competing treatments on the principal outcome of interest is sufficient to determine which treatment *should* be used in a particular population or individual patient (14). Altered self-perception, illness behavior, economic costs, treatment side effects, and other problems (most or all of which are generally ignored in randomized clinical trials) may have a significant impact on a person's life and well-being. Consequently, even if the COMS randomized clinical trial of enucleation versus iodine-125 plaque radiotherapy shows one treatment to be "significantly" better than the other in terms of the principal outcome event rate (an outcome that I believe to be highly unlikely), that result will not provide sufficient justification for physicians to eliminate the "worse treatment" from the therapeutic armamentarium and insist that all patients undergo the "better treatment." If enucleation should prove better, can that result be extrapolated to other methods of irradiation? Would anyone infer from such a result that patients should not be treated by charged particle radiotherapy, cobalt-60 plaques, ruthenium-106 plaques, surgical resection of the tumor, hyperthermia, or other potentially eye-preserving therapies? The answer, of course, is "no." The best treatment for the individual patient must take into account that patient's perception of the probable quality of life after the intervention as well as the scientific evidence of the relative beneficial effects of one treatment over the other (14,15).

## Conclusion

I hope that my comments on randomized clinical trials and the COMS have been enlightening. It should be clear by now that I am a strong proponent of well-conceived and well-designed randomized clinical trials. It should also be apparent, however, that I do not believe the "randomized clinical trial" to be the correct answer to every question about relative therapeutic effectiveness in clinical medicine. Whether you agree or disagree with my viewpoint, I trust that you will at least recognize that my criticisms of the COMS are not frivolous but are based on what I believe to be the correct scientific interpretation of currently available information. Despite my decision not to support the COMS, however, I urge all interested ophthalmologists to acquaint themselves with that study, judge for themselves whether or not its design is scientifically valid and ethical, and then decide whether or not to participate in or support that study.

*References*


1. May WW: The composition and function of ethical committees. *J Med Ethics* 1:23–29, 1975.
2. Peto R, Pike MC, Armitage P, et al: Design and analysis of randomized clinical trials requiring prolonged observation of each patient. I. Introduction and design. *Br J Cancer* 34:585–612, 1976.
3. Simon RM: Design and conduct of clinical trials, in DeVita VT, Hellman S, Rosenberg SA (eds): *Cancer. Principles & Practice of Oncology,* ed 2. Philadelphia, Lippincott, 1985, pp 329–350.
4. Feinstein AR: *Clinical Epidemiology. The Architecture of Clinical Research.* Philadelphia, Saunders, 1985, pp 683–718.
5. Altman DG: Misuse of statistics is unethical, in Gore SM, Altman DG (eds): *Statistics in Practice.* London, British Medical Association, 1982, pp 1–2.
6. Fine SL: Do I take the eye out or leave it in? *Arch Ophthalmol* 104:653–654, 1986.
7. Manschot WA, van Strik R: Is irradiation a justifiable treatment of choroidal melanoma? An analysis of published results. *Br J Ophthalmol* 71:348–352, 1987.
8. Seddon JM, Gragoudas ES, Albert DM, et al: Comparison of survival rates for patients with uveal melanoma after treatment with proton beam irradiation or enucleation. *Am J Ophthalmol* 99:282–290, 1985.
9. Straatsma BR, Fine SL, Earle JD, et al: The Collaborative Ocular Melanoma Study Research Group. Enucleation versus plaque irradiation for choroidal melanoma. *Ophthalmology* 95:1000–1004, 1988.
10. Augsburger JJ, Gamel JW, Sardi VF, et al: Enucleation vs cobalt plaque radiotherapy for malignant melanomas of the choroid and ciliary body. *Arch Ophthalmol* 104:655–661, 1986.
11. Lommatzsch PK: Results after β-irradiation (106Ru/106Rh) of choroidal melanoma. 20 years' experience. *Br J Ophthalmol* 70:844–851, 1986.
12. Adams KS, Abramson DH, Ellsworth RM, et al: Cobalt plaque versus enucleation for uveal melanoma: comparison of survival rates. *Br J Ophthalmol* 72:494–497, 1988.
13. Gore SM: Assessing methods—art of significance testing, in Gore SM, Altman DG (eds): *Statistics in Practice.* London, British Medical Association, 1982, pp 70–72.
14. Forrow L, Wartman SA, Brock DW: Science, ethics, and the making of clinical decisions. Implications for risk factor intervention. *JAMA* 259:3161–3167, 1988.
15. Angell M: Patients' preferences in randomized clinical trials. *N Engl J Med* 310:1385–1387, 1984.

## Epidemiologic Aspects of Uveal Melanoma

Egan KM, Seddon JM, Glynn RJ, Gragoudas ES, Albert DM (Massachusetts Eye and Ear Infirmary, Boston; Harvard Med School)
*Surv Ophthalmol* 32:239–250, January–February 1988                    6–1

Uveal melanoma is an uncommon malignancy with a high rate of metastasis. It is the most frequent primary intraocular malignancy and the only primary intraocular disease of adults that can be fatal. The annual age-adjusted incidence of ocular melanoma is the United States using data from 1969 to 1971 is 6 cases per 1 million population. Other surveys of primarily white populations yield similar incidence rates (table).

Uveal melanoma, most often diagnosed in the sixth decade, is somewhat more common in males. Apart from sporadic reports of family clusters, it is not considered to be inherited. Sunlight, which causes cutaneous melanoma, has been proposed as an environmental risk factor; both diseases are rare in nonwhite races. However, rates of uveal melanoma have not been increasing over time, in contrast to cutaneous melanoma, and they do not vary by latitude. Further case-control studies should help to establish whether sunlight induces uveal melanoma. Objective measures of solar exposure are more accurate than self-reports.

Studies of whether ocular melanocytosis and oculodermal melanocytosis dispose to uveal melanoma could help to show whether uveal melanoma is one manifestation of a generalized melanocytic dysfunction. The small male excess of disease and exposures in the workplace, such as those exposed to welding arcs, deserve further study.

▶ The authors summarize incidence data on posterior uveal melanomas comprehensively and comment on the evidence for and against various hereditary and environmental factors in the etiology of this uncommon primary ocular malignancy. All ophthalmologists interested in the subject of posterior uveal

---

### Incidence Rates of Uveal Melanoma Reported for Various Populations

| | | | Rate (Incidence $\times 10^6$) | |
| Author | Population | Interval | With iris | Without iris |
|---|---|---|---|---|
| Shammas (1977) | Iowa (USA) (whites only) | 1969–1971 | 5.6 | 4.9 |
| Kurland (1987) | Rochester and Olmstead County, Minnesota (USA) | 1935–1974 | 6.7 | 6.0 |
| Egan (1987) | New England (USA) | 1984–1985 | — | 6.5 |
| Ganley (1973) | Washington County, MD (USA) | 1956–1965 | — | 6.6 |
| Raivio (1977) | Finland | 1953–1973 | 5.0 | — |
| Birdsell (1980) | Alberta, Canada | 1967–1976 | 6.0 | 5.5 |
| Jensen (1963) | Denmark | 1943–1952 | 7.4 | 7.1 |
| Abrahamsson (1983) | Swedish west coast | 1956–1975 | — | 7.2 |
| Mork (1961) | Norway | 1953–1960 | *8.0 | — |

*Primary anatomical site unavailable in this series.
(Courtesy of Egan KM, Seddon JM, Glynn RJ, et al: *Surv Ophthalmol* 32:239–250, January–February 1988.)

malignant melanoma should be completely familiar with the information contained in this paper.—J.J. Augsburger, M.D.

---

**Interval-by-Interval Cox Model Analysis of 3680 Cases of Intraocular Melanoma Shows a Decline in the Prognostic Value of Size and Cell Type Over Time After Tumor Excision**
Gamel JW, McLean IW, Greenberg RA (Univ of Louisville; Armed Forces Inst of Pathology, Washington, DC)
*Cancer* 61:574–579, Feb 1, 1988       6–2

Large intraocular melanomas are thought to have a worse prognosis than small ones, and those with a significant epithelioid cell component appear to have a worse prognosis than spindle cell tumors. In a series of 3,680 patients undergoing excision of a uveal melanoma from 1927 to 1979, there were 1,178 deaths ascribed to the tumor during 20 years after excision. The Cox statistical model was used to evaluate various prognostic factors.

A single-term analysis showed a decline over time in the Cox coefficients and their associated $t$ values. The prognostic value of largest tumor dimension and Callender cell type decreased significantly over time. The decline was similar whether coded deaths included those from all causes or those from melanoma only. Coefficients of 2-term models showed a time-related decline similar to that found through the interval-by-interval single-term analysis. Regression analysis indicated a substantial negative correlation of both largest tumor dimension and Callender cell type with log survival time.

By criteria of largest tumor dimension and Callender cell type, melanoma-related deaths and survivors are more difficult to distinguish at later than at earlier intervals. There seems to be some degree of actual decrease in the predictive value of these parameters over time after tumor excision. If the decline continues to the point of statistical insignificance, further follow-up may not yield more useful insights into the benefit of a particular treatment.

▶ The authors' observations that tumor size and melanoma cell type decrease in value as predictors of the length of survival after treatment until death from metastatic uveal melanoma may be pertinent to the design of prospective clinical studies of uveal melanoma management. The decrease in predictive value of these parameters over time suggests that, if short-term (within 5 years) follow-up fails to show any substantial difference in posttreatment survival rates, longer follow-up of the same patient groups is also unlikely to demonstrate a difference.—J.J. Augsburger, M.D.

---

**DNA Cell Cycle Studies in Uveal Melanoma**
Char DH, Huhta K, Waldman F (Univ of California, San Francisco)
*Am J Ophthalmol* 107:65–72, January 1989       6–3

Although most eyes with uveal melanoma that are treated with radiation are retained, the mean tumor shrinkage is only 40% and relatively few tumors are reduced to a flat scar. Irradiated uveal melanomas usually contain viable-appearing cells, although there is little if any evidence of mitotic activity. After intravenous injection of bromodeoxyuridine 1 hour before surgery, DNA synthesis was estimated in 29 patients. Eleven eyes were studied after primary enucleation and there were 5 ciliochoroidectomy tumor specimens. Five eyes were given 20 Gy of photon irradiation for 5 days before enucleation. Eight others received helium ion therapy and required enucleation for complications of treatment. Most specimens were fixed in 10% formalin and processed conventionally.

Flow cytometric analysis showed more melanoma cells in DNA synthesis in tumors not given ionizing radiation. The mean bromodeoxyuridine count in nonirradiated tumors was 79.5, compared with 0.8 for irradiated tumors. In no case could long-term, rapidly growing tissue culture cell lines be established. Explants from 7 nonirradiated tumors did remain viable for up to 15 passages. Two of 5 samples from tumors treated with 20 Gy of pre-enucleation radiation were maintained for 3 passages and 7 passages, respectively.

Uveal melanoma cell cycling is suppressed by irradiation, and exposed cells are less able to form expanded explants. Morbidity from in vivo bromodeoxyuridine studies is minimal, but there are a number of potential limitations to this assay. Use of the assay and fine-needle aspiration biopsy may help to identify successfully irradiated tumors.

▶ The techniques described by the authors are certainly innovative extensions of flow cytometry and fine-needle aspiration biopsy in patients with a posterior uveal melanoma. General clinical application of these methods, however, does not appear likely in the near future.—J.J. Augsburger, M.D.

---

## Comparison of Transillumination and Histologic Slide Measurements of Tumor Diameter in Uveal Melanoma

Polivogianis L, Seddon JM, Glynn RJ, Gragoudas ES, Albert DM (Massachusetts Eye and Ear Infirmary, Boston; Harvard Med School)
*Ophthalmology* 95:1576–1582, November 1988                6–4

---

Tumor size is an important prognostic factor in uveal melanoma. It is measured by ocular transillumination in patients who receive proton beam irradiation and histologically after enucleation. These methods were compared by measuring tumor diameter by transpupillary or transscleral transillumination in 45 consecutive, nonfixed eyes that were processed in the laboratory. In 40 evaluable cases the largest diameter of the tumor in contact with the sclera was measured.

The mean largest tumor diameter by transillumination was 16.1 mm, compared with 13.2 mm for histology. There was good correlation between the 2 methods. It is possible that highly elevated tumors produce a shadow that leads to overestimation of their size on transillumination.

Tissue shrinkage may lead to an underestimate of size on histologic study. Standard sectioning along the pupil-optic nerve axis does not always yield the largest diameter. These results reflect measurements of transillumination after enucleation and may differ from clinical measurements.

Survival studies must address the issue of measuring tumor size so that outcomes after various treatments can be compared in a meaningful way.

▶ The authors reported a "good correlation" between their in vitro transillumination estimates and pathologic measurements of the basal dimensions of posterior uveal melanomas. Of course, such a result is not surprising to anyone who has a modicum of familiarity with linear regression analysis. Because the authors were simply measuring the same variable by 2 different methods, one would expect them to have found a strong correlation (just as one would expect a strong correlation between intraocular pressure measurements obtained by 2 different methods). The more impressive result was the magnitude of the difference between the mean values of the largest linear basal tumor diameter estimated by the 2 methods, with the transillumination estimates tending to be substantially larger.

The authors did not address the fact that the relationship between clinical estimates and pathologic measurements may not be linear over the full range of tumor encountered clinically. The reader should recognize that a survival comparison between groups of enucleated as opposed to irradiated patients is likely to be biased in favor of the irradiated patients if tumor size is estimated by transillumination in the irradiated group and by pathology measurements in the enucleated group. One must also realize that transillumination performed in vivo may given substantially less reproducible and reliable estimates of tumor basal size than did the in vitro transillumination method described in this article.—J.J. Augsburger, M.D.

---

**Prognostic Significance of Histopathological Parameters in Malignant Melanoma of the Choroid as Determined by pTNM Classification**
Göllnitz R, Lommatzsch PK (Karl-Marx-Universität Leipzig, East Germany)
*Klin Monatsbl Augenheilkd* 192:296–301, 1988         6–5

---

A retrospective histopathologic prognostic factor analysis was carried out on a group of 376 patients who underwent enucleation for choroidal malignant melanoma during a 22-year period. Potential prognostic factors, assessed by review of the histologic specimens, included tumor size (categorized by the 1982 tumor/node/metastasis (TMN) classification), melanoma cell type, degree of pigmentation, extent of scleral invasion, and mitotic activity.

Cell type was the most important predictor of length of survival until death from metastatic melanoma. Patients with spindle cell tumors had a substantially better prognosis than did those with mixed or epithelioid cell type lesions. Other significant predictors of length of survival included degree of pigmentation (patients with a more heavily pigmented tumor having the less favorable prognosis), extent of scleral invasion (patients with extrascleral extension of tumor having the less favorable prognosis), and tumor size (patients with larger tumors having the less favorable prognosis). Mitotic activity had no significant prognostic value. Most of these findings are consistent with information reported previously.

▶ The results of this analysis are, by and large, consistent with what has been reported elsewhere by many authors over the years. I would criticize the authors, however, for using the TNM classification for specification of tumor size. Various authors in the United States have repeatedly shown that the largest linear tumor dimension, measured either histopathologically or clinically, seems to be a much more reliable predictor of a tumor's malignant potential than is its size classified according to the TNM system.—J.J. Augsburger, M.D.

---

**Melanoma Arising De Novo Over a 16-Month Period**
Sahel JA, Pesavento R, Frederick AR Jr, Albert DM (Harvard Med School; Ophthalmic Consultants of Boston)
*Arch Ophthalmol* 106:381–385, March 1988                                    6–6

---

A patient was seen with a large uveal melanoma arising from the posterior choroid in an eye that had been free of any lesion 16 months previously.

Woman, 71, had late-onset diabetes and systemic hypertension. Bilateral laser iridotomies had been done because of narrow angle glaucoma. Fundus examination showed microangiopathic diabetic retinopathy with extensive macular edema. Argon laser photocoagulation was done in the left perimacular region. Cataracts progressed in both eyes. An apparent mass was found in the right eye 16 months after last examination, with a secondary retinal detachment. Enucleation was carried out, and microscopy confirmed a mixed-type choroidal melanoma with invasion of the optic disk. Electron microscopy confirmed a predominance of epithelioid cells admixed with spindle cells. The largest tumor diameter at the base was 19 mm and the height was 11 mm.

Calculations indicated that the average doubling time of this melanoma is 64 days at most, corresponding to the lowest found by Gass in a series of growing melanomas. This is consistent with the high mitotic index observed. It is likely that, as is the case with cutaneous melanomas, uveal melanomas can arise either from preexisting nevi or melanosis or de novo. In the latter case the tumor could induce a nevus-like configuration by flattening of normal uveal melanocytes or modification of tumor cells when infiltrating the sclera; the configuration could also represent a secondary proliferative effect of the malignancy.

▶ The fact that a sizable malignant melanoma developed within a previously normal region of the choroid during a 16-month interval indicates that, at least in some patients, the rate of tumor growth may be very rapid. Furthermore, this case illustrates the fact that all choroidal melanomas do not develop from preexistent, clinically identifiable choroidal nevi.—J.J. Augsburger, M.D.

**Internal Eye Wall Resection in the Management of Uveal Melanoma**
Peyman GA, Charles H (Louisiana State Univ)
*Can J Ophthalmol* 23:219–223, 1988                                      6–7

A technique of transvitreal tumor resection was carried out in 20 patients with presumed uveal melanoma. Patients were selected for this procedure if the tumor extended to within 1–2 disks diameters of the optic nerve without evidence of nerve invasion on ophthalmoscopy, computed tomography, or magnetic resonance imaging; if complete assessment found no metastatic disease; and if the patient's general health allowed for 3–4 hours of general anesthesia.

About 1 month before surgery patients underwent peripheral scatter retinal photocoagulation. Hypotensive anesthesia was used to prevent choroidal or retinal hemorrhage during resection. The surface and underside of the tumor, the resection bed, and the margins of the tumor were treated with argon endophotocoagulation, intraocular neodymium:yttrium/aluminum/garnet laser energy, or intraocular carbon dioxide laser light. The tumor was then dissected, and complete vitrectomy and air-fluid exchange were done. Silicone oil was then injected into the vitreous cavity through a sclerotomy. An encircling band was placed around the globe in all cases.

Follow-up ranged from 2 to 37 months. In all patients the retina was completely attached at the last examination. Visual acuity ranged from 20/40 to hand movements; 9 patients had acuity of 20/400 or better. At the last examination no metastatic disease or local recurrence had developed in any of the 15 patients in whom malignant melanoma was confirmed histologically.

Internal eye wall resection offers advantages in removing uveal melanoma within 2 disk diameters of the optic nerve head and in eliminating residual suspect tissue along the margins of previously resected sites. Intraoperative complications in this series were uncommon.

▶ The technique described by the authors is extraordinarily complex and limited in scope. Because of its complexity, it seems unlikely ever to become a common method of managing choroidal and ciliary body melanomas. The authors appear to believe that the visual results are good, but I am not particularly impressed; the visual results of substantially less aggressive interventions (e.g., charged particle irradiation and episcleral plaque radiotherapy) tend to be much better than the reported results of this procedure, at least in the first few years after treatment. Although ophthalmic oncologists from several centers have reported diagnostic error rates in the range of approximately 2% to 5% during the past decade, the authors of this paper had a diagnostic error rate of 25%.—J.J. Augsburger, M.D.

### Preliminary Results on Phosphorus-31 Nuclear Magnetic Resonance Evaluation of Human Uveal Melanoma in Enucleated Eyes

Kolodny NH, Gragoudas ES, D'Amico DJ, Seddon JM, Minichiello M, Murphy EJ, Albert DM (Massachusetts Eye and Ear Infirmary, Boston; Harvard Med School; Massachusetts Inst of Technology, Cambridge; Wellesley College)
*Ophthalmology* 95:666–673, May 1988                                    6–8

Many lesions, both benign and malignant, can simulate choroidal melanoma on ophthalmoscopy. Magnetic resonance (MR) spectroscopy with $^{31}$P is a means of diagnosing these lesions and is also able to assess tumor viability and the response to treatment. Spectra were recorded from 8 enucleated human eyes suspected of having uveal melanoma. The eyes were maintained at 4 C in tissue culture medium, and MR spectra were obtained within 10 minutes using a 2-turn $^{31}$P surface coil.

Magnetic resonance spectroscopy distinguished choroidal melanomas from normal ocular structures. Significant peaks in tumor spectra were produced by the phosphodiesters glycerol 3-phosphoryl ethanolamine and glycerol 3-phosphorylcholine, and the phosphomonoesters phosphorylethanolamine and phosphorylcholine.

The $^{31}$P MR spectral features of choroidal melanoma differ significantly from those of normal ocular structures. Spectra can be recorded in less than 10 minutes using a small surface coil adjacent to the eye. Attempts are underway to extend this approach to tumors in the human eye in vivo.

▶ The real value of MR spectroscopy will probably not be known for many years. However, this paper brings us up to date about the current status of this potentially useful "high-tech" diagnostic test.—J.J. Augsburger, M.D.

### Risk of Nonocular Cancer Among Retinoblastoma Patients and Their Parents: A Population-Based Study in Denmark, 1943–1984

Winther J, Olsen JH, Brown PdN (Danish Cancer Society, Aarhus; Danish Cancer Registry, Copenhagen; Aarhus Univ Hosp, Denmark)
*Cancer* 62:1458–1462, Oct 1, 1988                                    6–9

Various studies have shown patients with genetic retinoblastoma to be at risk for new primary cancers developing later in life, although the reported risk has varied greatly. The incidence and time trend of retinoblastoma were determined in a national population of 4–5 million persons from 1943 to 1984. The relative risk of second primary tumors also was determined.

In survivors, retinoblastoma had been treated with radiotherapy or surgery alone; chemotherapy was not administered. Retinoblastoma was identified in 175 patients during the study period. The overall cumulative incidence rate was therefore 5.5 cases per 100,000 liveborn children. A borderline significant 40% increase in incidence throughout the period studied was noted. Twenty-five patients died of metastases related to the retinoblastoma; in 3 of the 150 survivors a new primary malignancy developed.

The expected number of new second primary tumors among survivors was 0.7, yielding a relative risk of 4.2. Two of the second cancers were diagnosed in the subgroup of genetic cases, compared with 0.13 expected tumors, which yields a relative risk of 15. No second primary cancers occurred in the field of irradiation among 47 patients given radiotherapy for retinoblastoma. Two of the second primary cancers occurred in the long bones of the limbs, yielding a relative risk of about 100. Fourteen cancers developed in 267 parents after the birth of an index child. The relative risk for fathers and mothers was 1.11 and 0.67, respectively.

The number of second primary nonocular cancers among survivors of retinoblastoma in this study was surprisingly low compared with previous findings. Chemotherapy applied in previously published series may be responsible for at least some of the substantially increased risks for second tumors in these patients.

▶ This paper presents some of the best information currently available concerning the risk of nonocular cancer in retinoblastoma survivors and their parents. Because the data in this paper are derived from a population-based group, the estimated risks of nonocular cancers developing as presented by these authors appear to be believable.—J.J. Augsburger, M.D.

---

**Retinoblastoma in Great Britain 1969–80: Incidence, Treatment, and Survival**
Sanders BM, Draper GJ, Kingston JE (Univ of Oxford; St Bartholomew's Hosp, London)
*Br J Ophthalmol* 72:576–583, 1988                                    6–10

---

Retinoblastoma comprises approximately 3% of all malignant tumors in children. A long-term follow-up study analyzed incidence and second primary tumors and examined trends in treatment. Patients with retinoblastoma diagnosed between 1969 and 1980 were observed for up to 17 years. Previous published data on patients with retinoblastoma diagnosed from 1962 to 1968 also were studied. Included were 431 children in England, Scotland, and Wales.

The overall incidence was 43.9 per million births, or 1 in 23,000 births. Slightly more than 60% of the tumors were unilateral, the incidences of unilateral and bilateral cases being 1 in 37,000 and 1 in 60,000 births, respectively. About 40% were genetic. The 3-year survival rate was 88%. Patients with bilateral tumors had a better survival rate than those with unilateral tumors for the first few years, but their long-term survival rate was lower because of later deaths from ectopic intracranial retinoblastoma or second primary neoplasms. Older children tended to have worse prognoses, and there was a significantly higher survival rate for boys than for girls. Children referred to units specializing in retinoblastoma treatment had a higher 3-year survival rate than those treated elsewhere. A trend toward more conservative treatment was noted. The use of chemotherapy is currently usually reserved for recurrences and metastases and for palliative treatment in terminal cases. Of the 5 children with second primary neoplasms, 3 died.

This study found the incidence of retinoblastoma to be similar to that found in earlier reports. No change in incidence over the period studied was observed, and there has been very little change in the already high 3-year survival rate for these patients.

▶ I believe that this paper contains the best currently available summary of the incidence of retinoblastoma and the management and survival of children afflicted by it. The authors' total of 431 cases accumulated over 11 years is impressive.—J.J. Augsburger, M.D.

---

**Incidence of Second Neoplasms in Patients With Bilateral Retinoblastoma**
Roarty JD, McLean IW, Zimmerman LE (Armed Forces Inst of Pathology, Washington, DC; Georgetown Univ)
*Ophthalmology* 95:1583–1587, November 1988                    6–11

---

Children who survive retinoblastoma are at increased risk of a second primary neoplasm developing, possibly because of a genetic mutation. The influence of radiation therapy has remained uncertain. To determine the effect of radiation therapy on the incidence of second nonocular tumors, the records of 215 patients with bilateral retinoblastoma were studied. All had an eye enucleated between 1922 and 1973. All were from the United States. The life-table method of analysis was used. The

Types of Second Tumors That Developed in 24 Retinoblastoma Survivors

| | No. of Tumors | | |
|---|---|---|---|
| Type of Tumor | Irradiated | Non-irradiated | Total |
| Osteogenic sarcoma | 4 | 1 | 5 |
| Chondrosarcoma | 1 | 0 | 1 |
| Sarcoma, spindle-cell type | 2 | 0 | 2 |
| Melanoma | 1 | 3 | 4 |
| Sebaceous carcinoma | 2 | 0 | 2 |
| Transitional cell carcinoma | 1 | 0 | 1 |
| Squamous cell carcinoma | 1 | 1 | 2 |
| Carcinoma, undifferentiated | 1 | 0 | 1 |
| Undifferentiated malignancy | 0 | 1 | 1 |
| Myxoma | 1 | 0 | 1 |
| Leukemia | 0 | 1 | 1 |
| Pinealoblastoma | 0 | 2 | 2 |
| Neuroblastoma | 0 | 1 | 1 |
| Glioma | 0 | 1 | 1 |
| Brain tumor, unknown type | 0 | 1 | 1 |
| Total | 14 | 12 | 26 |

(Courtesy of Roarty JD, McLean IW, Zimmerman LE: *Ophthalmology* 95:1583–1587, November 1988.)

inclusion of only bilateral cases ensured that all patients had a mutation.

Eighty-seven patients died of retinoblastoma and 26 second tumors developed in 24 patients (table). Second tumors developed in 4.4% of patients in the first 10 years of follow-up, in 18.3% after 20 years, and in 26.1% after 30 years. The 30-year cumulative rate was 35.1% in 137 patients who were given radiation therapy and 5.8% in the 78 who were not so treated. In patients who received radiation, second tumors developed both within and outside the field of treatment, but the rate was more than three-fold greater within the field of treatment. Sarcomas accounted for 38% of the secondary tumors; cutaneous melanoma was the next most common neoplasm.

Carriers of the retinoblastoma gene have an increased risk of second tumors, and those who receive radiation therapy are especially vulnerable. The finding that osteosarcoma occurs in carriers of the retinoblastoma gene at about the same age as it does in the general population suggests that carriers may have decidedly increased rates of gastrointestinal, lung, and breast cancers when they approach the usual age of onset of these neoplasms. Recent data suggest that chemotherapy also may increase the risk of second tumors in carriers of the retinoblastoma gene.

▶ This article is important for three reasons. First, it provides clinicians with a reasonable actuarial estimate of the cumulative risk that a survivor of germinal retinoblastoma will have an independent, nonretinoblastoma malignancy within 20–30 years. In the discussion section of the article the authors compare and contrast their results in this regard with the published results of other investigators. Second, they address the issue of radiotherapy's effect on the long-term incidence of nonretinoblastoma malignancies within and outside the field of irradiation. Third, this article raises the question of a possible additional adverse effect of chemotherapy on the cumulative risk of a second malignancy developing.—J.J. Augsburger, M.D.

---

**Prediction of the Risk of Hereditary Retinoblastoma, Using DNA Polymorphisms Within the Retinoblastoma Gene**

Wiggs J, Nordenskjöld M, Yandell D, Rapaport J, Grondin V, Janson M, Werelius B, Petersen R, Craft A, Riedel K, Liberfarb R, Walton D, Wilson W, Dryja TP (Massachusetts Eye and Ear Infirmary, Boston; Karolinska Inst, Stockholm; Children's Hosp, Boston; Royal Victoria Infirmary, New Castle upon Tyne, England; Augenklinik der Universität, Munich; et al)

*N Engl J Med* 318:151–157, Jan 21, 1988                                6–12

---

From 30% to 40% of retinoblastoma patients have an inherited predisposition to the tumor, as well as to other cancers, determined by a locus within the q14 band of chromosome 13. Retinoblastoma develops in 80% to 90% of persons having any of a variety of mutant alleles at this locus. There is evidence that sporadic cases arise from retinal cells having somatic mutations at the same genetic locus.

Recently, DNA sequences corresponding to the retinoblastoma gene were cloned. One approach to diagnosis requires cloned DNA fragments from the retinoblastoma gene that detect DNA polymorphisms, or restriction-fragment-length polymorphisms (RFLPs). The use of RFLPs allowed predictions of the cancer risk to be made in 19 of 20 kindreds with hereditary retinoblastoma. In 18 kindreds marker RFLPs were consistently associated with the mutation disposing to retinoblastoma; in the 19th kindred there may be a lack of cosegregation of the DNA polymorphisms within the gene and the site of the mutation predisposing to tumor. There is some uncertainty about the clinical diagnosis in a key member of this kindred.

It appears feasible to use DNA polymorphisms to determine the risk of retinoblastoma. The analysis relies on RFLPs identified within the retinoblastoma locus and, in a few families, on identification of deletions involving the locus presumably representing loss-of-function mutations. Certain key family members—typically, affected parents—must be heterozygous for the DNA polymorphism evaluated. About 95% of families are informative in this way. Rarely, the marker DNA polymorphism and the site of the causative mutation are not inherited together.

▶ The use of DNA RFLPs appears to be a significant advance over karyotype analysis in the prediction of hereditary retinoblastoma. With further experience and improvement in this genetic technique, ophthalmologists may have a reliable method of prenatal screening for retinoblastoma in families in which one of the parents-to-be is a retinoblastoma survivor.—J.J. Augsburger, M.D.

---

**Frozen Section of the Optic Nerve in Retinoblastoma Surgery**
Karcioglu ZA, Haik BG, Gordon RA (Tulane Univ)
*Ophthalmology* 95:674–676, May 1988                                    6–13

---

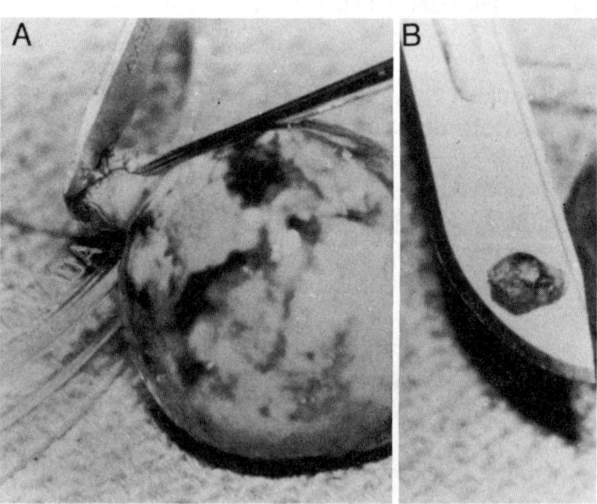


Fig 6–1.—**A,** sectioning of the optic nerve stump for frozen section from an enucleated globe with retinoblastoma. **B,** resection margin of the optic nerve stump obtained for frozen section is shown on the scalpel blade. (Courtesy of Karcioglu ZA, Haik BG, Gordon RA: *Ophthalmology* 95:674–676, May 1988.)

Frozen section study of the optic nerve margin is important when retinoblastoma is removed, because extension of tumor into the optic nerve may lead to involvement of the subarachnoid space. Resection margins were examined by frozen section in 7 consecutive enucleations for retinoblastoma. In all eyes the tumor mass covered the optic disk either partially or totally. A transverse section of the most distal part of the optic nerve was sampled (Fig 6–1). Three cryosections from different depths were taken at the time of sectioning.

Tumor tissue was present at the resection margin in 2 of 7 cases. The length of the positive stumps was 7 mm and 9 mm, respectively. Additional segments of nerve were resected in these cases, and examination of the specimens was negative for tumor. Gross examination of the nerve stump was not informative.

Frozen section study of optic nerve specimens are useful in detecting tumor at the resection margin in cases of retinoblastoma. The procedure takes less than 5 minutes, and its great advantage is that the results are available in the operating room. If the margin is free of tumor, orbital recurrence is most unlikely.

▶ The actual benefit of this frozen section technique is not really apparent. Most children who have tumor extension more than a few millimeters into the optic nerve will probably ultimately die of disseminated retinoblastoma, regardless of whether the cut end of the nerve does or does not have identifiable tumor cells on frozen section analysis. Thus this technique may actually give the surgeon a false sense of security regarding the likelihood of cure.—J.J. Augsburger, M.D.

---

**Pigmented Ocular Fundus Lesions in the Inherited Gastrointestinal Polyposis Syndromes and in Hereditary Nonpolyposis Colorectal Cancer**
Traboulsi EI, Maumenee IH, Krush AJ, Giardiello FM, Levin LS, Hamilton SR (Johns Hopkins Univ; Georgetown Univ)
*Ophthalmology* 95:964–969, July 1988                                 6–14

---

Multiple patches of congenital hypertrophy of the retinal pigment epithelium (CHRPE) have been described in a large number of kindreds with Gardner's syndrome. They have also been noted in 4 patients from 2 families with familial adenomatous polyposis coli. Families with hereditary nonpolyposis colorectal cancer have not been examined for the presence of pigmented ocular fundus lesions. Such lesions were studied in 3 different forms of hereditary gastrointestinal polyposis and in hereditary nonpolyposis colorectal cancer.

In all, 174 members of 33 families were examined. Congenital hypertrophy of the retinal pigment epithelium was noted in at least 1 member of 23 families with Gardner's syndrome but was not found in 3 families with familial polyposis coli, 4 families with hereditary nonpolyposis colorectal cancer, or 3 families with Peutz-Jeghers syndrome.

This study found patches of CHRPE exclusively in patients with and family members at risk for Gardner's syndrome. Extraintestinal lesions in this syndrome include osteomas, especially skull and mandible epidermoid cysts, odontomas, lipomas, fibromas, and desmoid tumors. Colon cancer develops in 100% of untreated patients.

▶ This paper helps to clarify the prognostic significance of characteristic pigmented fundus lesions in individuals with the gene for Gardner's syndrome. The presence of bilateral, multifocal hypertrophic lesions of the retinal pigment epithelium in a member of a kindred with Gardner's syndrome is reliably predictive that that individual also has colonic polyposis and will have carcinoma of the colon.—J.J. Augsburger, M.D.

# 7  Pathology

## New Developments in the Genetics of Retinoblastoma

Ralph C. Eagle, Jr., M.D.
*Department of Pathology, Wills Eye Hospital, Philadelphia, Pennsylvania*

Retinoblastoma is presently the focus of intensive basic research that has led to major advances in our understanding of the retinoblastoma gene and molecular events involved in the pathogenesis of this important childhood malignancy. The ophthalmologist should be familiar with these exciting and important new developments because he or she is the physician who diagnoses and treats most patients with this intraocular tumor and is responsible for providing genetic counseling. These important new concepts are not only elegant and intellectually satisfying; if properly understood, they can actually aid the clinician in his recall and understanding of retinoblastoma's varied clinical manifestations.

Clinically, several variants of retinoblastoma are recognized. Approximately 5% to 10% of cases are familial. They are inherited in what appears to be a classic Mendelian autosomal dominant fashion. Affected patients transmit the disease to approximately one half of their offspring, in whom bilateral and multifocal tumors typically develop.

The great majority of retinoblastomas are sporadic; these tumors are diagnosed in patients who have no family history of retinoblastoma. Three fourths of these sporadic tumors are thought to arise from somatic mutations that occur in a single retinal cell. Such patients have a normal genotype and cannot transmit the tumor to their offspring. The remaining fourth of sporadic tumors are new familial cases. They result from germinal mutations and are transmissible.

In addition, retinoblastoma develops in a small number of patients with karyotypically obvious deletions in the long arm of chromosome 13. Although rare, the association of retinoblastoma with the 13 q-syndrome is important, because it provided the initial evidence that the gene responsible for retinoblastoma was located on a segment of the long arm of chromosome 13.

Using powerful new molecular genetic techniques, researchers subsequently isolated and cloned the RB or retinoblastoma gene and determined its sequence of constituent base pairs. Using the genetic code, the amino acid sequence of the RB gene's protein product was predicted. It subsequently was shown that this protein (called p105-RB) resides in the nucleus of the cell. This nuclear phosphoprotein has DNA binding activity and appears to play a critical role in the expression of other cellular genes and in limiting cellular proliferation. Similar proteins are found in all vertebrate species.

The RB gene causes retinoblastoma in an indirect manner. Tumors develop when the normal gene has been lost or inactivated. Healthy cells normally contain 2 functional copies of the RB gene that direct the synthesis of a "double dose" of the p105 RB suppressor protein that functions at the molecular level to limit cellular proliferation. If this suppressor protein is absent or nonfunctional, a cell undergoes malignant transformation. This occurs when both copies of the retinoblastoma suppressor gene in that cell have been lost, damaged, or inactivated. Genetic misadventures or mutations that lead to gene loss or damage generally occur during cellular division. The estimated mutation rate for the RB gene is $10^{-7}$; hence, on average, in every 10 million cellular divisions 1 copy of the retinoblastoma gene is lost or inactivated.

Carriers of familial retinoblastoma are heterozygous for the RB gene. A carrier's genotype includes a wild type or functional RB gene that directs the synthesis of a single dose of p105-RB suppressor protein. The other gene has been lost, damaged, or inactivated. The single dose of suppressor substance in a heterozygous cell generally is sufficient to prevent malignant transformation. If the single remaining healthy RB gene in a cell is also lost or damaged, however, that cell will become cancerous because no suppressor substance is present. As noted, this happens approximately once in every $10^7$ mitoses. It has been estimated that 100 million $(10^8)$ mitoses are involved in the growth and development of the neurosensory retina. Because the spontaneous mutation rate of the retinoblastoma gene is 10 times smaller, it is therefore highly probable that the retina of a heterozygous carrier harbors at least 1 cell with no suppressor protein that will spawn a retinal tumor. Furthermore, because $10^8$ mitoses are involved in the growth and development of each retina, it is equally probable that a retinoblastoma will develop in the fellow eye. These probability estimates are also consistent with the development of multiple or multifocal retinoblastomas in patients with familial disease.

Clinically, approximately two thirds of patients with familial retinoblastomas actually have bilateral tumors. If a patient has bilateral retinoblastoma one must assume that he or she harbors the retinoblastoma gene and is capable of transmitting the tumor to offspring. Unfortunately, the opposite is not true. Because the penetrance of the RB gene is only 80%, the remaining patients with familial retinoblastoma have unilateral tumors.

The heterozygous nature of retinoblastoma gene carriers readily explains why familial retinoblastoma appears to be inherited in an autosomal dominant fashion. When a heterozygous carrier mates with a normal individual, 50% of the expected offspring are heterozygous carriers: RB rb (carrier) $\times$ RB RB (normal) = 50% RB RB and 50% RB rb.

The great majority of retinoblastomas arise sporadically in patients who have no family history of the disease. Three fourths of these sporadic tumors are thought to result from the loss or inactivation of both RB genes in a single retinal cell. The probability of this occurrence is the product of the spontaneous mutation rate, i.e., $10^{-7} \times 10^{-7}$ or $10^{-14}$. Because the probability of dual gene inactivation occurring in more than

1 retinal cell is so exceedingly minute, sporadic somatic retinoblastomas are invariably unilateral and unifocal. Patients who have sporadic somatic retinoblastomas have a normal genotype and therefore they cannot transmit the tumor to their offspring.

The remaining one fourth of sporadic retinoblastomas, which are termed "sporadic germinal" tumors, are new familial cases. They result from RB gene loss during gametogenesis or conception. Like familial cases, affected individuals with sporadic germinal tumors are heterozygous, and they typically have bilateral and multifocal retinoblastomas that are transmissible.

These new genetic concepts explain other hitherto puzzling features of retinoblastoma. For example, why is retinoblastoma predominantly a tumor of early childhood? Although retinoblastoma has been reported in adults, the tumor is extremely rare after age 4 years; in 90% of these patients the diagnosis is made by age 3. The explanation is simple: Adult retinal neurons do not divide. In fact, most mitotic activity in the retina actually ceases by birth. Because cytogenetic misadventures that cause gene loss or inactivation generally occur during cellular division, neoplastic transformation in older patients is extremely unlikely. The theory also suggests why bilateral hereditary tumors also develop at an earlier age (average, 12 months) than unilateral sporadic tumors (average, 23 months). In familial cases only 1 gene must be inactivated, and this presumably takes less time.

Patients who harbor the retinoblastoma oncogene are also at risk for the development of second primary tumors elsewhere in the body. It has been estimated that a survivor of bilateral retinoblastoma has a 20% to 50% chance of a second primary tumor developing within 20 years. These second tumors include osteogenic sarcoma of the orbit and femur. Survivors of bilateral retinoblastoma are reported to have a 500-fold increase in the incidence of osteogenic sarcoma of the femur. From the ophthalmic standpoint, one of the most interesting secondary tumors is a retinoblastoma-like tumor of the pineal gland called pineoblastoma. This association, which is termed "trilateral retinoblastoma," should be suspected clinically when a survivor of bilateral retinoblastoma has headache or papilledema.

Recent evidence suggests that the retinoblastoma gene may play a fundamental role in other nonocular cancers. Inactivation of the RB gene has been observed in other types of tumors including some breast and lung carcinomas, synovial sarcomas, and other soft tissue sarcomas. The retinoblastoma gene is also thought to mediate the oncogenic effects of certain tumor viruses. It was shown recently that the protein produce of the retinoblastoma gene forms stable complexes with the oncoproteins of SV40 and adenovirus that produce tumors in animals, and the E7 oncoprotein of human papillomavirus. The latter virus has been strongly linked to cervical cancer. It is thought that the retinoblastoma gene product is inactivated by the binding of these viral oncoproteins, thus mimicking the loss of the RB 1 gene as seen in the genetic predisposition to retinoblastoma.

In the future, clinical ophthalmology is certain to derive new practical benefits from this research. Diagnostic tests will soon be available that will allow the ophthalmologist to accurately identify carriers of the retinoblastoma gene. Novel therapeutic strategies for treatment of retinoblastoma such as gene replacement therapy are another possibility. Unlike conventional cytotoxic therapy, gene therapy would be based on permanent correction of the underlying defect in the tumor cells. This proposal is not as far-fetched as it sounds. Huang and associates already have used retrovirus carriers to insert normal retinoblastoma genes back into retinoblastoma cells growing in tissue culture. In contrast to untreated control retinoblastoma cells, cells treated with the retinoblastoma gene grow very slowly in culture, undergo a marked change in their morphology, and do not produce tumors when injected into nude mice.

*Suggested Reading*

Benedict WF, Murphree AI, Banerjee A, et al: Patient with chromosome deletion: Evidence that the retinoblastoma gene is a recessive cancer gene. *Science* 219, 1983.

Dyson N, Howley PM, Münger K, et al: The human papilloma virus-16 E7 oncoprotein is able to bind to the retinoblastoma gene product. *Science*. In press.

Godbout R, Dryja TP, Squire J, et al: Somatic inactivation of genes on chromosome 13 is a common event in retinoblastoma. *Nature* 304:451, 1983.

Huang HJS, Yee JK, Shew JY, et al: Suppression of the neoplastic phenotype by replacement of the RB gene in human cancer cells. *Science* 242:1563, 1988.

Lee WH, Bookstein R, Hong FD, et al: Human retinoblastoma susceptibility gene: Cloning, identification, and sequencing. *Science* 235:1394, 1987.

Lee WH, Shew JY, Hong FD, et al: The retinoblastoma susceptibility gene encodes a nuclear phosphoprotein associated with DNA binding activity. *Nature* 329:642, 1987.

Lee WH, Bookstein R, Lee YHP: Studies on the human retinoblastoma susceptibility gene. *J Cell Biochem* 38:213, 1988.

Murphree AL, Benedict WF: Retinoblastoma: Clues to human oncogenesis. *Science* 223:1028, 1984.

Roarty JD, McLean IW, Zimmerman LE: Incidence of second neoplasms in patients with bilateral retinoblastoma. *Ophthalmology* 95:1583, 1988.

---

**Idiopathic Senile Macular Hole: Its Early Stages and Pathogenesis**
Gass JDM (Univ of Miami)
*Arch Ophthalmol* 106:629–639, May 1988

7–1

Biologic changes in the prefoveal vitreous cortex cause it to shrink. This initially produces anterior traction detachment of the retina, first in the foveolar area and then in the foveal region. Shortly afterward, tangential traction and foveolar hole formation take place. Impending hole formation is characterized by biomicroscopic findings of a yellow spot or ring in the center of the fovea and loss of the foveal depression. There is no evidence of separation of the vitreous from the foveal retina. Most eyes with these changes progress to hole formation, but in some cases

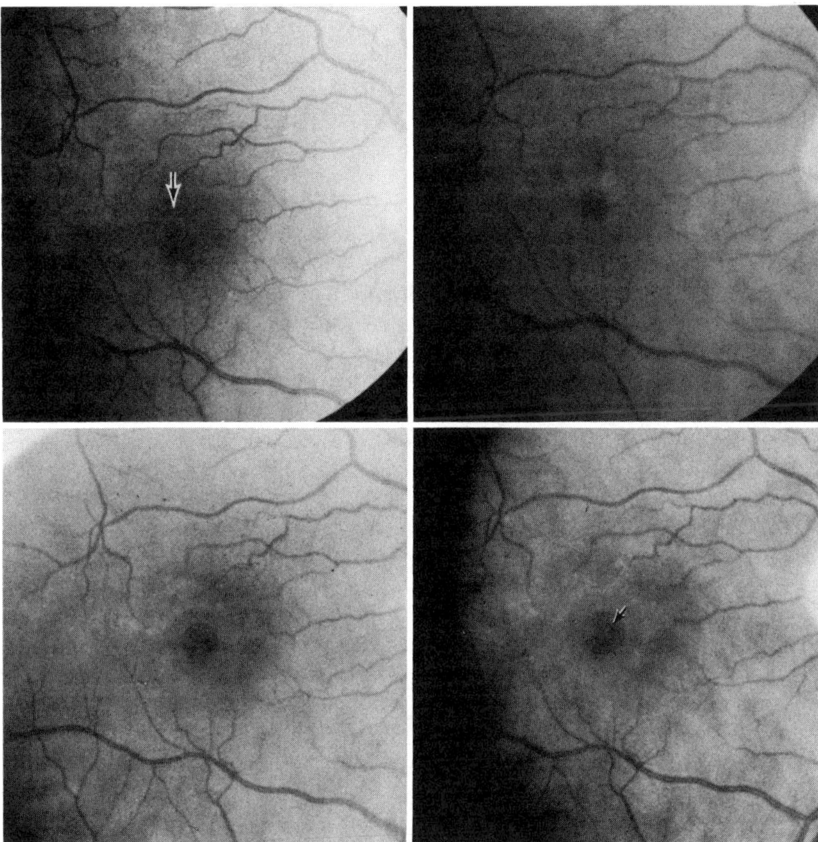

**Fig 7–1.**—Right eye of patient. **Top left,** May 18, 1966, stage 1B, foveal detachment with yellow ring *(arrow)*. **Top right,** August 15, 1967, stage 2 eccentric hole extending clockwise from 9 to 3 o'clock positions. White spot is artifact. **Bottom left,** August 2, 1968, stage 2 hole extending clockwise from 7 to 5 o'clock positions. **Bottom right,** August 1971, stage 3 hole with operculum *(arrow)*. (Courtesy of Gass JDM: *Arch Ophthalmol* 106:629–639, May 1988.)

there is spontaneous separation of the vitreous without hole formation. Foveal reattachment is seen in these cases. There sometimes is a pseudo-operculum with 1 or more lamellar holes or facets (Fig 7–1).

The most reliable features of impending hole formation are a yellow foveolar spot or ring, loss of the foveal depression, radiating retinal striae, and the absence of vitreofoveal separation associated with recent loss of visual function. In most such eyes a full-thickness macular hole develops (Fig 7–2) within several weeks or months. Theoretically, either surgical peeling or partial peeling and segmentation of the prefoveal vitreous cortex might prevent macular hole formation in eyes with early changes.

▶ Don Gass does it again. This paper, one of a series of outstanding contributions, shows how keen observational skills and thoughtful analysis of carefully

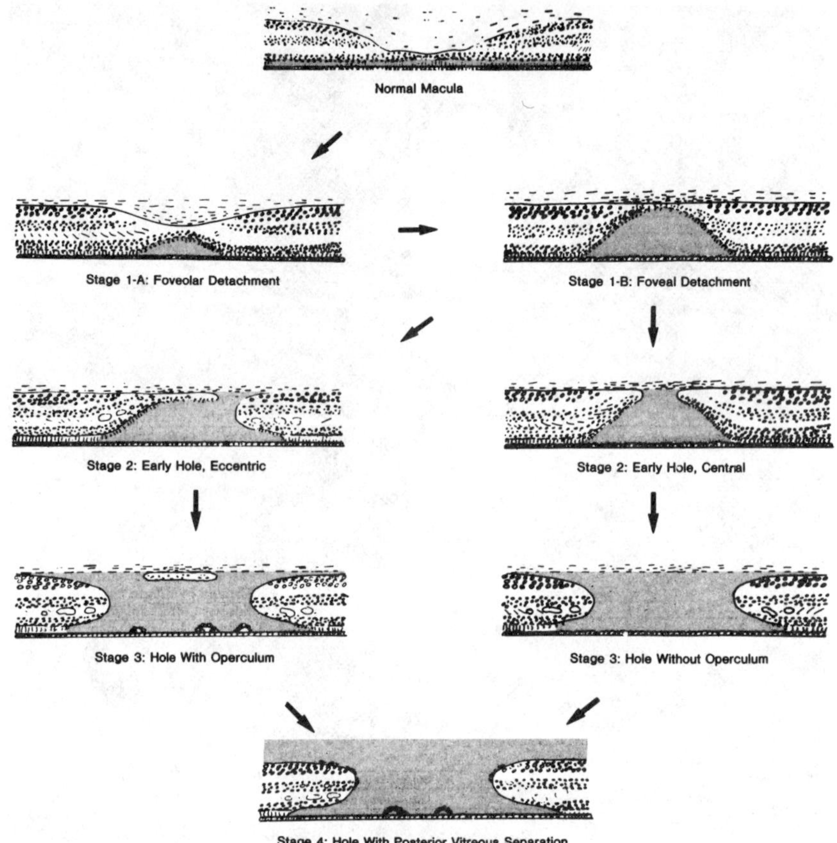


**Fig 7–2.**—Diagram of presumed stages of development of idiopathic senile macular hole. (Courtesy of Gass JDM: *Arch Ophthalmol* 106:629–639, May 1988.)

documented clinical data can lead to a cogent hypothesis that can elucidate the pathogenesis of a previously enigmatic disorder. Not merely elegant and intellectually satisfying, Dr. Gass' hypothesis has potential therapeutic applicability. If idiopathic senile macular holes are spawned, as Dr. Gass contends, by tractional foveal detachment, then expeditious vitreoretinal surgery could possibly forestall progression to bilateral blindness. It remains to be seen if vitreoretinal surgeons will have the courage to attempt such potentially disastrous prophylactic surgery on the remaining healthy eyes of predisposed patients.—R.C. Eagle, Jr., M.D.

## Decentration of Flexible Loop Posterior Chamber Intraocular Lenses in a Series of 222 Postmortem Eyes

Hansen SO, Tetz MR, Solomon KD, Borup MD, Brems RN, O'Morchoe DJC, Bouhaddou O, Apple DJ (Univ of Utah)
*Ophthalmology* 95:344–349, March 1988

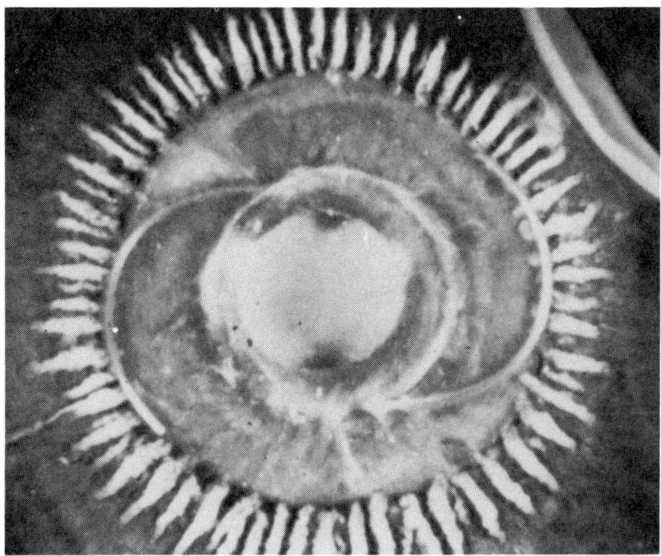

Fig 7–3.—Gross photograph from behind of a postmortem eye showing capsular fixation of a short or modified C-loop posterior chamber intraocular lens. The loops conform nicely to the circular configuration of the capsular bag, and the optic is well centered. (Courtesy of Hansen SO, Tetz MR, Solomon KD, et al: *Ophthalmology* 95:344–349, March 1988.)

Examinations were made of 222 eyes obtained at autopsy that contained posterior chamber intraocular lenses. Optic decentration was analyzed in relation to lens type, loop fixation site, and implant duration. Only flexible loop lenses, including J-loop, modified J-loop, and C-loop styles, were included.

The site of loop fixation was the only factor that significantly influenced the amount of optic decentration of the intraocular lens. One third of the lenses had symmetric bag/bag fixation (Fig 7–3), whereas 18% exhibited symmetric sulcus/sulcus fixation. The rest had asymmetric bag/uveal fixation, 18 of these 108 lenses having zonular or pars plana fixation. Asymmetric loop placement clearly caused the most decentration; about 60% of such lenses had decentration values of at least 0.8 mm. Three fourths of symmetrically fixated lenses were decentered by 0.6 mm or less, thereby retaining a more effective optical zone. Only one symmetrically fixated lens decentered more than 2 mm.

Bag/bag fixation of a posterior chamber intraocular lens provides less decentration than sulcus/sulcus fixation or bag/uveal fixation. There is little reason not to attempt capsular fixation in all cataract patients in whom preexisting disease and intraoperative complications are absent. Current technology allows capsular fixation to be achieved consistently.

▶ In nearly one half of the eyes in this large autopsy series, only 1 loop of a posterior chamber intraocular lens was present in the capsular bag. The authors optimistically state that current technology allows surgeons to achieve capsular fixation consistently if they attempt to do so. It will be interesting to see if the incidence of symmetric capsular fixation will increase in future studies.—R.C. Eagle, Jr., M.D.

## Histopathology of Traumatic Corneal Rupture After Radial Keratotomy

Binder PS, Waring GO III, Arrowsmith PN, Wang C (Sharp Cabrillo Hosp, San Diego; Emory Univ; Arrowsmith Eye Research Found, Nashville)
*Arch Ophthalmol* 106:1584–1590, November 1988                    7–3

Radial keratotomy involves a series of radial incisions in the paracentral and peripheral cornea that weaken the cornea and bow the incised area forward. The central cornea flattens as a result, decreasing its refrac-

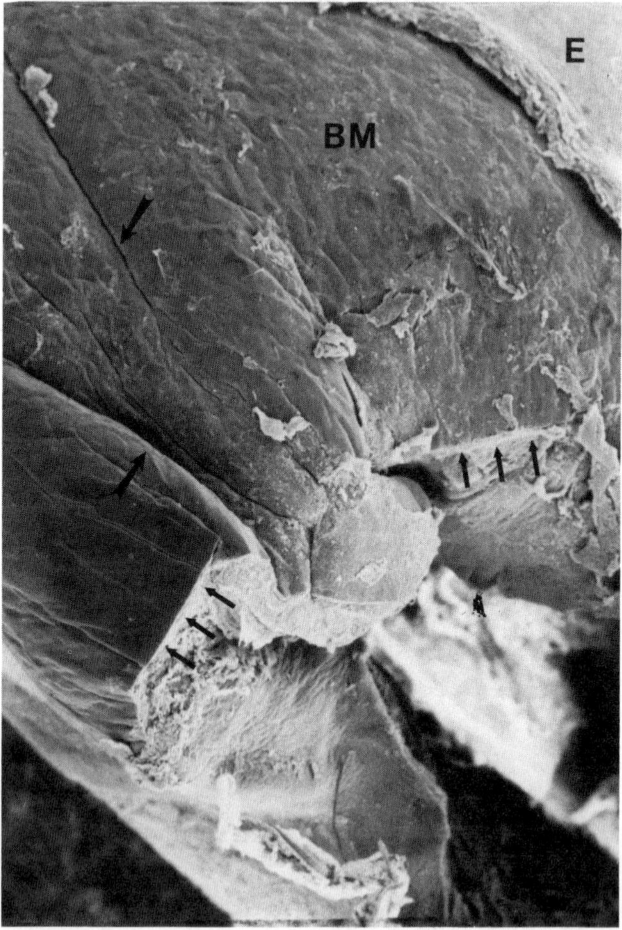


Fig 7–4.—Corneal surface of right eye of man aged 27 years. Rupture occurred along 2 opposing incisions across optical zone, leaving 2 other incisions *(large arrows)* intact. *Small arrows* mark sharp edge of Bowman's layer. *E*, epithelium; *BM*, Bowman's membrane. Scanning electron microscopy; original magnification, ×44. (Courtesy of Binder PS, Waring GO III, Arrowsmith PN, et al: *Arch Ophthalmol* 106:1584–1590, November 1988.)

tive power. The operated-on cornea is at increased risk of rupturing after blunt injury to the globe.

Two patients with 3 affected eyes had undergone technically successful radial keratotomy and subsequently incurred blunt trauma to the eyes in motor vehicle accidents. Injury occurred 1 year and 2 years after keratotomy. The corneas ruptured along the lines of the keratotomy scars (Fig 7–4). One patient required penetrating keratoplasty and recovered acuity of 20/50. The other patient died, but had he lived, his ocular injuries would have required extensive care to regain vision. Some wounds were healing, but others extended through the full corneal thickness and caused wide scarring.

After radial keratotomy, the epithelium remains in many wounds for a

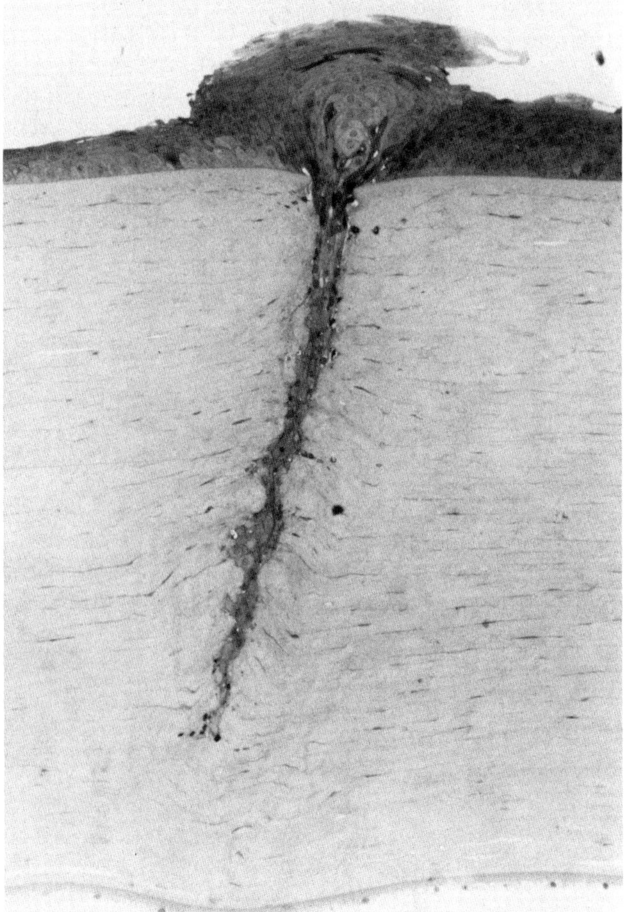

**Fig 7–5.**—Left eye of same patient as in **Fig 7–4.** Multiple epithelial cells formed elevated facet just above incision. Epithelial cells also line entire depth of wound and probably migrated there after traumatic reopening of wounds. Minimal fibroblastic activity was seen around incision. Hematoxylin-eosin; original magnification, ×200. (Courtesy of Binder PS, Waring GO III, Arrowsmith PN, et al: *Arch Ophthalmol* 106:1584–1590, November 1988.)

long time (Fig 7–5), as do active fibroblasts. Once healing is complete, there is a stromal scar matrix that helps to bind together the 2 sides of the wound. Corneal wounds never become as strong as the original cornea, and persons having radial keratotomy should know of the hazards of a weakened cornea. Prolonged use of steroids should be avoided after this operation.

## Heterogeneity in Macular Corneal Dystrophy

Edward DP, Yue BYJT, Sugar J, Thonar EJ-MA, SunderRaj N, Stock EL, Tso MOM (Univ of Illinois, Chicago; Rush-Presbyterian-St Luke's Med Ctr, Chicago; Northwestern Univ; Eye and Ear Inst of Pittsburgh)
*Arch Ophthalmol* 106:1579–1583, November 1988                    7–4

Macular corneal dystrophy is an infrequent disorder that is inherited as an autosomal recessive trait. There are poorly defined corneal opacities and a ground-glass stromal haze, which are usually noted at puberty. The opacities eventually coalesce to impair vision. The deposits represent a fibrillogranular material that is found intracellularly in stromal keratocytes and extracellularly among the stromal collagen fibers. This material is thought to be an abnormal proteoglycan.

Corneal buttons were obtained from 12 patients with an established

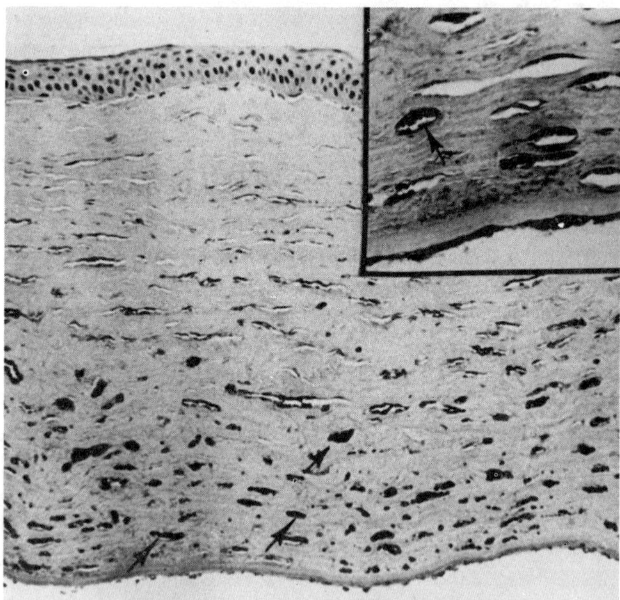

Fig 7–6.—Corneal section showing positive staining with monoclonal antibody J-19. There is positive staining *(arrows)* in posterior stromal keratocytes (avidin-biotin peroxidase; original magnification, ×480). Inset shows positive staining of keratocytes and endothelium (avidin-biotin-peroxidase; original magnification, ×1,920). (Courtesy of Edward DP, Yue BYJT, Sugar J, et al: *Arch Ophthalmol* 106:1579–1583, November 1988.)

clinical diagnosis of macular corneal dystrophy. All specimens stained positively with colloidal iron. Four reacted with monoclonal antibody that recognized sites on the sulfated keratan sulfate molecule (Fig 7–6), but 8 corneas did not react with any of the 4 antibodies used. One of 7 patients had a normal serum level of keratan sulfate; this patient and 2 others had positive corneal immunostaining. The clinical features could not be related to the histochemical or ultrastructural findings.

Apparently, there are variants of macular corneal dystrophy characterized by different forms of keratan sulfate in the cornea. The clinical and pathologic findings are similar in the various forms.

**Paraproteinemic Crystalline Keratopathy**
Ormerod LD, Collin HB, Dohlman CH, Craft JL, Desforges JF, Albert DM (Harvard Med School; Retina Found; Tufts Univ; Univ of New South Wales, Kensington, Australia)
*Ophthalmology* 95:202–212, February 1988                    7–5

Paraproteinemic crystalline keratopathy, present for at least 16 years, was found in a patient with monoclonal gammopathy of unknown significance. Such keratopathy is an infrequent complication of multiple myeloma and other plasma cell dyscrasias. The present patient had an IgG kappa monoclonal gammopathy and recurrent uveitis. Extensive changes involved all layers of the cornea. Diffuse, small, polymorphic aggregates were associated with a stromal haze. Histochemical staining was unrevealing, but there was extensive immunohistochemical labeling for IgG, kappa, and also lambda. Ultrastructural study showed deposits in all corneal cells and paracrystalline deposits with internal banding in the basal epithelium only. Keratocytes and endothelial cells were damaged and reduced in number. The disease recurred in a corneal graft.

The natural course of crystalline keratopathy usually is prolonged, suggesting that corneal disease occurs in a subgroup of patients with more indolent disease than typical myeloma. All cases except those associated with Waldenström's macroglobulinemia have involved IgG monoclonal proteins; most have had kappa Ig light chains. Paraproteinemic crystalline keratopathy may involve the anterior stroma, all of the stroma diffusely, or the posterior stromal region, depending on whether it arises from the tears, limbal vessels, or aqueous humor, respectively. Diffuse stromal disease has been described in 5 patients in association with recurrent anterior uveitis. The deposits probably represent metabolic products of the monoclonal immunoglobulin.

The differential diagnosis of crystalline keratopathy includes cystinosis, gout, chronic renal failure, hypercalcemia, lipid keratopathy, the crystalline dystrophies of Schnyder and Bietti, as well as the keratopathies of multiple myeloma and related states.

▶ Monoclonal gammopathy of unknown significance denotes the presence of a monoclonal protein in serum or urine without evidence of multiple myeloma, macroglobulinemia, or a related disease. The workup of the patient who has corneal crystals should include serum protein electrophoresis to rule out a plasma cell dyscrasia.—R.C. Eagle, Jr., M.D.

**Cryotherapy for Conjunctival Primary Acquired Melanosis and Malignant Melanoma: Experience With 62 Cases**
Jakobiec FA, Rini FJ, Fraunfelder FT, Brownstein S (Manhattan Eye, Ear & Throat Hosp; Columbia-Presbyterian Med Ctr, New York; Oregon Health Sciences Univ, Portland; McGill Univ, Montreal)
*Ophthalmology* 95:1058–1070, August 1988                                    7–6

Several reports have described the advantages of using cryotherapy instead of extensive conjunctivectomy and exenteration in the management of flat conjunctival primary acquired melanosis (PAM) and nodular malignant melanoma. In the largest series of premalignant and malignant melanocytic tumors of the conjunctiva treated to date, 62 patients underwent some combination of cryotherapy and surgery and were observed for an average of 3.3 years.

Ten patients had PAM with atypia but without a nodule of melanoma; 30 had unifocal malignant melanoma with or without focal or diffuse PAM, and 22 had multinodular/multicentric melanoma with and without PAM. Of the 10 patients with PAM and atypia, invasive nodules of malignant melanoma did not develop. A second treatment was needed to control the disease in 4 of the 10 patients with extensive or diffuse lesions; 1 patient continued to have mild persistent disease. Of the 30 patients in the second group, 27 remained free of recurrence after 1 treatment and 2 are asymptomatic after 2 treatments. One patient with a thick nodule required parotidectomy and radical neck dissection because of cervical metastases after recurrence in the conjunctival sac. Of the 22 patients in the third group, only 2 did not have recurrent disease after 1 treatment. Of those who received multiple treatments, 7 remained recurrence free for at least 2 years, had regional or distant metastases, 4 required exenteration, and 8 died.

Conjunctival adjunctive cryotherapy avoided exenteration in extensive lesions of pure PAM and in unifocal melanoma, but even after multiple therapies, multinodular malignant melanoma had a 45% rate of metastasis. Metastasis was related to PAM sine pigmento, to the nodule location, to thickness or depth of nodule invasion, and to intralymphatic spread in the conjunctival sac. There were no metastases among patients with strictly limbal nodules or among 5 patients with invasive nodules composed of spindle cells in part or in toto.

Therapeutic success in this spectrum of melanocytic proliferations is closely correlated with the clinical extent of disease when initiating definitive treatment.

▶ This important study underscores the need to diagnose and treat PAM, an in situ form of conjunctival melanoma, in the early stages before the vertical growth phase of invasive malignant melanoma ensues. Once multiple nodules of malignant melanoma have developed, all therapeutic modalities, including cryotherapy and orbital exenteration, are unable to prevent the development of fatal metastatic disease in nearly half of the patients.—R.C. Eagle, M.D.

## Choroidal Melanoma With Pigment Dispersion in Vitreous and Melanomalytic Glaucoma

El Baba F, Hagler WS, de la Cruz A, Green WR (Johns Hopkins Med Inst, Baltimore; Piedmont Hosp, Atlanta)
*Ophthalmology* 95:370–377, March 1988                    7–7

A black man aged 39 years underwent enucleation because of poor vision, ocular pain, and intractable glaucoma secondary to a choroidal tumor. Diagnostic vitrectomies done 11 months and 7 months before enucleation failed to demonstrate the tumor. The histologic diagnosis was necrotic malignant melanoma of the choroid with melanocytoma cells, extensive pigment dispersion throughout the eye, and melanomalytic glaucoma. Pigmented macrophages and free melanin were seen in the trabecular meshwork and Schlemm's canal, the anterior and posterior chambers (Fig 7–7), the vitreous, along the inner retinal surface and optic nerve head, and within the sclera and episclera at sclerotomy sites.

The pathogenesis of tumor necrosis is not understood. Extreme dispersion of pigment and pigmented macrophages was noted in the present patient, suggesting that the macrophages may have had a role in mediating tumor necrosis. Inflammation and tumor necrosis may delay the diagnosis of melanoma for some time. Open-angle glaucoma in the present pa-

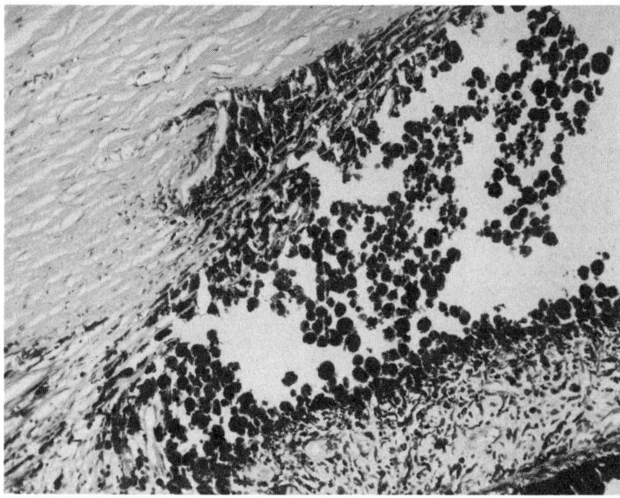

**Fig 7–7.**—Pigmented macrophages along anterior surface of the iris and in the angle, intratrabecular spaces, and Schlemm's canal (hematoxylin-eosin; original magnification, ×180). (Courtesy of El Baba F, Hagler WS, de la Cruz A, et al: *Ophthalmology* 95:370–377, March 1988.)

tient was a result of mechanical blockage of the trabecular meshwork by pigment-laden macrophages (melanomalytic glaucoma). A similar complication has been found in necrotic melanocytomas.

▶ Posterior uveal melanomas usually induce secondary closed-angle glaucoma through iris neovascularization or pupillary block. In this case, the open angle was occluded by macrophages that had engulfed pigment liberated by a necrotic choroidal tumor.—R.C. Eagle, Jr., M.D.

## Quantitation of Tumor Seeding From Fine Needle Aspiration of Ocular Melanomas

Glasgow BJ, Brown HH, Zargoza AM, Foos RY (Univ of California, Los Angeles)
*Am J Ophthalmol* 105:538–546, May 1988                                     7–8

Clinicians may hesitate to perform intraocular aspiration biopsy in some cases because of potential complications, such as tumor seeding in the needle path, with resultant local or systemic implantation of malignant cells. Recent studies have not shown tumor recurrence or metastases to result from intraocular fine-needle aspiration biopsy (FNAB). To decrease the risk of extraocular seeding, a transocular route has been recommended so that tumor-free tissue and fluids cleanse the needle of adherent tumor cells. A reliable way to identify fine-needle tracts in enucleated eyes was sought in 22 fine-needle (30-gauge) aspirations done in eyes enucleated after the clinical diagnosis of melanoma.

Cytologic preparations were assessed for adequacy of material. Needle tracts were evaluated for tumor implanation. All needle tracts were identified with a scleral marking method. The number of tumor cells in tracts of direct transcleral aspiration was then compared with those in tracts of indirect aspiration that traversed the anterior chamber or vitreous.

Cellular material taken with 30-gauge needles was sufficient for the diagnosis of malignant melanoma in all but 1 eye. Sixty-seven percent of 21 FNAB tracts and 53% of 15 indirect aspiration tracts contained tumor cells, but the number of tumor cells was less than that associated with tumor growth in experimental models. Indirect aspiration tracts contained significantly fewer cells than did direct tracts.

Transocular aspiration resulted in significantly fewer tumor cells within tracts than did direct aspiration and 3 orders of magnitude fewer than needed for tumor implant survival. These findings support the theory that transocular aspiration is less likely to lead to extraocular seeding than direct aspiration is.

▶ The major indication for intraocular FNAB is differentiation between choroidal amelanotic melanoma and metastatic carcinoma when clinical findings and studies are inconclusive. In my experience, examination of needle tracts in globes enucleated after FNAB rarely discloses melanoma cells. Retinoblastoma can cause extensive seeding, however. I believe that eyes with suspected

retinoblastoma should be biopsied only in exceptional circumstances, if at all.—
R.C. Eagle, M.D.

---

**Primary Intraocular Lymphoma (Ocular Reticulum Cell Sarcoma) Diagnosis and Management**
Char DH, Ljung B-M, Miller T, Phillips T (Univ of California, San Francisco)
*Ophthalmology* 95:625–630, May 1988                                              7–9

---

Primary intraocular lymphoma can present as an isolated ocular tumor, or may involve both the globe and the central nervous system (CNS). Older patients usually are affected. Chronic diffuse uveitis or vitritis unresponsive to steroids often leads to misdiagnosis. Eventually, most patients die of CNS lymphoma.

Twenty patients (mean age, 61 years) with intraocular lymphoma had ocular or CNS disease. Eighteen patients had bilateral ocular involvement. Irregular yellowish or white retinal or chorioretinal lesions were noted in 16 patients. Vitreous biopsy can establish the diagnosis in more than 95% of cases. Characteristic cytologic findings included irregular nuclear contour, nuclear lobation, coarse and irregular chromatin, and the presence of nucleoli. Mitoses were seen occasionally; inflammatory cells were infrequent. Six of 9 specimens analyzed were null cell lymphomas, two were polyclonal, and 2 were probable T cell neoplasms. Lymphocyte marker analysis is of limited use in this setting.

More than 1 vitreous biopsy may be necessary to diagnose intraocular lymphoma, as in 3 of the present patients. Many of these patients may be salvaged by brain and ocular irradiation plus intrathecal chemotherapy. Patients with gross, symptomatic CNS involvement generally do poorly. The proper management of patients with ocular involvement alone remains uncertain.

▶ The long-term survival of patients with primary intraocular lymphoma treated by Dr. Char and his associates in recent years has increased dramatically. The authors suggest that their therapeutic success results largely from a regimen that combines ocular and CNS irradiation and intrathecal chemotherapy. An additional factor contributing to lengthened survival may be early diagnosis. As clinicians have become increasingly familiar with this rare intraocular malignancy, the average interval between onset of symptoms and diagnosis has decreased markedly.—R.C. Eagle, Jr., M.D.

---

**Hemangioblastoma of the Optic Nerve: Report of a Case and Review of Literature**
Nerad JA, Kersten RC, Anderson RL (Univ of Iowa; Univ of Cincinnati; Univ of Utah)
*Ophthalmology* 95:398–402, March 1988                                            7–10

---

Vascular tumors of the optic nerve are rare.

Woman, 26, with von Hippel-Lindau disease had an optic nerve hemangioblastoma that caused total loss of vision. The initial diagnosis was made by incisional biopsy. Progressive proptosis and loss of light perception developed before lateral orbitotomy for excision. Clinically and radiographically, the lesion resembled an optic nerve meningioma or glioma.

The optic disk may be involved by hemangioblastoma on occasion, but involvement of the retrobulbar optic nerve is rare. A review of data on 7 reported patients showed that progressive proptosis and optic atrophy were present initially, with visual loss ensuing. In some cases the tumor was a solitary finding, whereas in others stigmata of von Hippel-Lindau disease eventually developed. The operative findings in 3 patients showed that the tumor grew directly from within the nerve rather than from the nerve sheath. Hemangioblastoma of the optic nerve steadily enlarges and finally causes marked visual dysfunction.

Incisional biopsy is indicated if good vision remains and the diagnosis is in doubt. When profound visual loss has occurred and there is significant proptosis, en bloc excision of the optic nerve and hemangioblastoma is indicated. If intracranial extension is suspected, transcranial orbitotomy with exploration of the optic chiasm is called for. Patients should be monitored for evidence of von Hippel-Lindau disease.

▶ Strictly speaking, the patient reported did not have von Hippel-Lindau disease. Although multiple cerebellar tumors (Lindau's disease) were present, the retinal angiomas described by von Hippel were not observed. Tumors in the retina, optic nerve, or cerebellum all display identical histologic features; they are hemangioblastomas, not capillary hemangiomas.—R.C. Eagle, Jr., M.D.

---

## Relationship Between Sympathetic Ophthalmia, Phacoanaphylatic Endophthalmitis, and Vogt-Koyanagi-Harada Disease

Chan C-C (Natl Eye Inst, Bethesda)
*Ophthalmology* 95:619–624, May 1988                    7–11

---

Both similarities and differences exist between sympathetic ophthalmia and phacoanaphylatic endophthalmitis, and between sympathetic ophthalmia and Vogt-Koyanagi-Harada (VKH) disease. Sympathetic ophthalmia usually occurs within 2 weeks to 2 months after penetrating injury that involves uveal tissue; 90% of these patients are seen within 1 year. Many eyes with sympathetic ophthalmia have the classic histopathologic changes of phacoanaphylatic endophthalmitis. The few histologic studies of VKH disease show similarities to sympathetic ophthalmia.

A spectrum may exist with the T cell-mediated disease, sympathetic ophthalmia at one end and the B cell-related immune complex disease of phacoanaphylatic endophthalmitis at the other. Sympathetic ophthalmia is a lymphokine release response with few inflammatory products and without necrosis. Phacoanaphylatic endophthalmitis is an antibody-antigen reaction with many inflammatory cells, chemotactic factors, and necrosis. In the center is VKH disease, also a T cell-mediated disorder but with a spontaneous onset. Many B lymphocytes and plasma cells are present, and the serum IgD is elevated. Retinal detachment is a feature of VKH disease.

Both sympathetic ophthalmia and VKH disease are treated by intensive topical and systemic steroids or other immunosuppressive medication. Cyclosporine A may be indicated, but renal toxicity must be kept in mind. The only means of preventing sympathetic ophthalmia is removal of the injured globe before the other eye is affected, but usually an attempt to save the injured eye is warranted. Surgical removal of remaining lens material is indicated in phacoanaphylatic endophthalmitis; topical steroids are used to limit ocular inflammation.

▶ Although an attempt usually should be made to save a severely traumatized eye, prevention remains the best "treatment" for sympathetic uveitis. The clinician must be careful not to let the availability of new technology and instrumentation cloud his clinical judgment. Enucleation is still the only operation that should be performed if a traumatized eye is hopelessly blind.—R.C. Eagle, Jr., M.D.

---

**Delayed Onset Sympathetic Ophthalmia**
McClellan KA, Billson FA, Filipic M (Sydney Eye Hosp, Woolloomooloo, New South Wales, Australia)
*Med J Aust* 147:451–454, Nov 2, 1987                           7–12

---

Sympathetic ophthalmia after a perforating ocular injury involving incarceration of uveal tissue rarely occurs within 2 weeks of injury but may develop any time afterward. Three such patients were seen up to 62 years after ocular injury. One patient had sympathetic ophthalmia that developed spontaneously 62 years after a shotgun pellet had penetrated an eye. The other 2 patients had surgery on a previously injured eye, followed by bilateral granulomatous panuveitis that developed after 1 week and 7 years, respectively. In all cases the interval from ocular injury to the development of sympathetic ophthalmia was at least 11 years.

Sympathetic ophthalmia that is unusually delayed after initial injury frequently develops in an eye that is phthisical or has clinical evidence of ongoing inflammation. The role of elective surgery in 2 of the described patients is uncertain. Sympathetic ophthalmia has occurred after surgery on an uninjured eye. Sympathetic uveitis may be seen more often as more attempts at secondary reconstructive surgery are made in severely injured eyes. This should dictate caution when reconstructive surgery is considered, and patients should be aware of the risk.

▶ According to classic clinical teaching, enucleation is the only operation that should be performed on a hopelessly blind eye. These reports of sympathetic uveitis that followed reconstructive surgery serve to underscore the wisdom of this dictum.—R.C. Eagle, Jr., M.D.

## The Expanding Ophthalmologic Spectrum of Lyme Disease

Aaberg TM (Emory Univ)
*Am J Ophthalmol* 107:77–80, January 1989                                        7–13

Lyme disease is an immune-mediated multisystem disorder characterized by erythema chronicum migrans, an expanding skin lesion, after a bite by *Ixodidae* ticks. The disease is caused by the spirochete *Borrelia burgdorferi*, which is transmitted by these ticks. Ocular disorders are seen at all stages of Lyme disease.

Conjunctivitis may occur in early Lyme disease. The presence of iridocyclitis, retinal vasculitis, optic perineuritis, and diffuse choroiditis have all been described. In the second stage when cardiac and neurologic involvement occurs, there may be cranial neuropathies including Bell's palsy or paresis of the third or sixth cranial nerve. Bilateral keratitis involving the superficial and deep corneal stroma has been noted at this stage. Arthritis and chronic neurologic symptoms develop, and patients at this stage may report decreased vision or diplopia.

Lyme disease at all stages responds to tetracycline or doxycycline. Children can be treated with penicillin V or amoxicillin.

Because the organism has now been isolated in most areas of the United States, ophthalmologists must maintain a clinical awareness of Lyme disease in patients who have been in endemic regions and have unusual forms of conjunctivitis, keratitis, iridocyclitis, retinal vasculitis, or disk edema.

## Cowden's Disease

Bardenstein DS, McLean IW, Nerney J, Boatwright RS (Armed Forces Inst of Pathology, Washington, DC; Haywood County Hosp, Clyde)
*Ophthalmology* 95:1038–1041, August 1988                                        7–14

In a number of conditions, skin lesions alert physicians to an inapparent, concurrent, or impending malignant process. Cowden's disease is one such entity that frequently affects periocular structures. This disease is a rare genodermatosis in which the most common mucocutaneous lesions are multiple facial trichilemmomas, acral keratoses, and oral papillomas. The disease is associated with increased rates of breast and thyroid cancer and benign tumors and hamartomas of multiple organ systems. Multiple facial trichilemmomas are pathognomonic and may appear as lesions on the eyelid and periorbital skin. These tumors are composed of large, pale, glycogen-rich epithelial cells surrounded centrally by a single layer of smaller palisaded cells. Small keratin-containing cysts and scattered mitotic figures are common.

Girl, 17 years, had multiple tender papular lesions on the upper eyelid. The lesions had been present for several months without change. Biopsy of 4 lesions was done. Two years after treatment by excision, 2 new lesions appeared on the same eyelid. Histopathologic analysis showed that each tumor was composed of large, pale, polyhedral cells in a lobular configuration. At the periphery of the lobules, palisading of the basal layer and a thickened basement membrane were noted. The tumors, which contained scattered mitotic figures and small keratin cysts, were interpreted as trichilemmomas.

Cowden's disease may be underdiagnosed. Because of its potentially serious association with internal malignant processes, the diagnosis must be early and accurate. In a patient with multiple small lesions of the periocular skin, more than 2 lesions should be excised to avoid missing the diagnosis of Cowden's disease. When a solitary trichilemmoma is diagnosed, a careful search for other lesions, followed by biopsy, is indicated.

▶ Other recently characterized syndromes with internal cancer and ocular signs include Torre's syndrome, with eyelid sebaceous adenomas, and Gardner's syndrome, in which multiple lesions resembling congenital hypertrophy of the retinal pigment epithelium are an ophthalmoscopic marker. Enlarged corneal nerves, submucosal neuromas, bilateral pheochromocytomas, and highly lethal medullary thyroid carcinomas occur in young patients who have multiple endocrine neoplasia syndrome type IIb. Rarely, patients with fatal visceral carcinomas have bilateral, diffusely infiltrating bland melanocysts of the uveal tract that cause secondary retinal detachment.—R.C. Eagle, M.D.

# 8 Pediatrics

## Is Congenital Esotropia Truly Congenital?

Leonard B. Nelson, M.D.
*Department of Pediatric Ophthalmology, Wills Eye Hospital, Philadelphia, Pennsylvania*

Congenital esotropia is defined as a large-angle, constant esotropia with onset during the first 6 months of life (1). It represents the most common form of strabismus, with an incidence of 1% to 2% (2,3) in the general population and accounting for 28% to 54% (4–7) of all esotropia. Even though Costenbader (4) introduced the term infantile esotropia in 1961 to describe this condition, the designation "congenital" is still widely used.

Attempts to define the onset of this condition are important for several reasons. If esotropia is congenital, i.e., existing at birth, the infant would have no chance of experiencing a normal binocular environment (8). This situation would agree with Worth's "sensory" concept (9) that congenital esotropia results from a deficit in a purported fusion center in the brain. According to his theory, the goal of restoring binocularity is considered hopeless because there is no way to provide this congenitally absent neural function. However, if the esotropia has a later onset, the abnormal condition would have been preceded by a period of normal binocular experience. This situation would support Chavasse's theory (10) that congenital esotropia is caused by mechanical factors and is potentially curable if the deviation can be eliminated in infancy.

In an attempt to learn whether esotropia is present at birth or develops later in infancy, Nixon and associates (11) systematically examined 1,219 normal alert infants in a newborn nursery. They were not able to identify a single infant with findings characteristic of congenital esotropia. The authors concluded that esodeviations similar to those found in congenital esotropia are not present at birth but most likely develop during the first few weeks to months of life (11). Because the patients in this series were not followed beyond the neonatal examination, the inclusion of infants in whom congenital esotropia may have developed could not be confirmed.

To study the development of strabismus in infancy prospectively, Archer and coworkers (12) evaluated the ocular alignment of 4,211 normal neonates and obtained follow-up examinations in a subset of them. They documented the development of the characteristic findings of congenital esotropia in three infants who were either orthotropic or exotropic at birth. The authors were not able to distinguish the normal infants from

This study was supported in part by a grant from Fight for Sight, Inc., New York, to the Fight for Sight Children's Eye Center of Wills Eye Hospital.

those with congenital esotropia on the basis of their neonatal motility findings. The esodeviations became constant between approximately 2 months and 4 months of age. Two infants who were noted to be moderately esotropic at 5 weeks of age were orthotropic within several months. Although there was an early predominance of exodeviations among the normal neonates, it resolved precipitously during the first 9 months of age. Therefore, even normal infants seem to have a period in which there is an anomalous binocular environment.

Although congenital esotropia is not found at birth, with rare exception, even advocates of the earliest surgery have found imperfect binocularity in their postoperative patients (1). Helveston and associates (13) reviewed their experience with 44 patients whose esotropia was confirmed during the first 6 months of life. Of 13 surgically aligned before age 12 months, none achieved stereopsis. In contrast, 12 of 31 operated on after 12 months could appreciate at least gross stereoscopic targets. These authors suggest that there may be 2 kinds of congenital esotropia: The first conforms to Worth's model and has no fusion potential; as a result, the eyes deviate in early infancy and early presentation and surgery are the rule. In the second kind, the concepts of Chavasse seem more appropriate; binocularity begins to develop but is overcome by motor factors later in infancy. Although surgery tends to be performed later in these patients, they are more likely to achieve some degree of stereopsis. Others have recently supported the concept that congenital esotropia probably comprises more than a single etiologic category (14).

Animal experimentation has demonstrated that the structural and functional integrity of binocular cells in the lateral geniculate nucleus and visual cortex requires early binocular experience (15–17). Crawford and coworkers (18) have shown that only a brief period of binocular dissociation in infant monkeys can cause a permanent loss of stereopsis despite subsequent prolonged periods of normal binocular visual input. However, there is no evidence from animal research that, in addition to stereopsis, other binocular functions (e.g., sensory and motor fusion) are similarly affected by abnormal visual experience early in life (8).

Two studies from Indiana University (11,12) document that the characteristic findings of congenital esotropia are not present at birth but develop during the first few months of life. Therefore, the term "infantile esotropia" might be used more appropriately to describe a constant large-angle esotropia with onset during the first 6 months of life.

*References*


1. Nelson LB, Wagner RS, Simon JW, et al: Congenital esotropia. *Surv Ophthalmol* 31:363–383, 1987.
2. Firedman Z, Neumann E, Hyams SW, et al: Ophthalmic screening of 38,000 children, age 1 to 2½ years, in child welfare clinics. *J Pediatr Ophthalmol Strabismus* 17:261–267, 1980.

3. Graham PA: Epidemiology of strabismus. *Br J Ophthalmol* 58:224–231, 1974.

4. Costenbader FD: Infantile esotropia. *Trans Am Ophthalmol Soc* 59:397–429, 1961.

5. Nordlow W: Age distribution of onset of estropia. *Br J Ophthalmol* 37:359–364, 1961.

6. Keiner GBJ: Physiology and pathology of the optomotor reflexes. I. Development of the optomotor reflexes. *Am J Ophthalmol* 42:233–251, 1956.

7. Seobee RG: Esotropia: Incidence, etiology, and results of therapy. *Am J Ophthalmol* 34:817–833, 1951.

8. von Noorden GK: A reassessment of infantile esotropia: XLIV Edward Jackson Memorial Lecture. *Am J Ophthalmol* 105:1–10, 1988.

9. Worth C: *Squint, Its Causes and Treatment.* Philadelphia, Blakiston, 1903.

10. Chavasse FB: *Worth's Squint.* Philadelphia, Blakiston, 1903.

11. Nixon RB, Helveston EM, Miller K, et al: Incidence of strabismus in neonates. *Am J Ophthalmol* 100:798–801, 1985.

12. Archer SM, Sondhi N, Helveston EM: Strabismus in infancy. *Ophthalmology* 96:133–137, 1989.

13. Helveston EM, Ellis FD, Schott J, et al: Surgical treatment of congenital esotropia. *Am J Ophthalmol* 96:218–228, 1983.

14. Friendly DS: Management of infantile esotropia, in Nelson & Wagner (eds): *Strabismus Surgery, Int Ophthalmol Clin* 25. Boston, Little Brown, 1985.

15. Hubel DH: Exploration of the primary visual cortex, 1955–1978. *Nature* 299:5515–5524, 1982.

16. Wiesel TN: Postnatal development of the visual cortex and the influence of environment. *Nature* 299:583–591, 1982.

17. von Noorden GK: Amblyopia: A multidisciplinary approach. Proctor lecture. *Invest Ophthalmol Vis Sci* 26:1704–1716, 1985.

18. Crawford JW, von Noorden GK, Meharg LS, et al: Binocular neurons and binocular function in monkeys and children. *Invest Ophthalmol Vis Sci* 24:491–495, 1983.

---

**Strabismus in Infancy**

Archer SM, Sondhi N, Helveston EM (Indiana Univ, Indianapolis)
*Ophthalmology* 96:133–137, January 1989                                            8–1

---

Data on ocular motility were obtained from more than 4,000 normal neonates to follow prospectively the development of strabismus in infancy. Congenital esotropia developed in 3 infants who were either orthotropic or exotropic at birth. Both infants who had pathologic exotropia were exotropic at birth but no more so than most normal neonates. The deviation in these children seems to develop at age 2–4 months, a time when normal infants become increasingly orthotropic (Fig 8–1).

There is a modestly increased risk of congenital esotropia in the small group of neonates with esodeviations. Esodeviation in the neonatal period is not, however, required for congenital esotropia to develop. In gen-

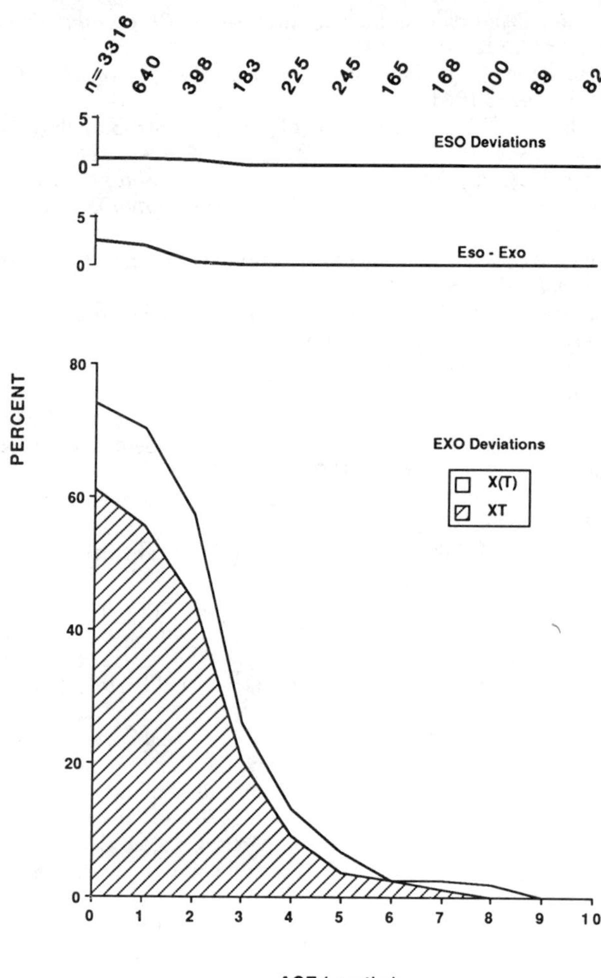


Fig 8–1.—Prevalence of various states of ocular alignment at various ages in normal population. Eight infants with specific pathologic strabismus diagnoses are not included. (Courtesy of Archer SM, Sondhi N, Helveston EM: *Ophthalmology* 96:133–137, January 1989.)

eral, normal infants and those with congenital esotropia or exotropia cannot be distinguished by the motility findings in the neonatal period. Abnormal motility usually is evident at about age 2–4 months.

## Management of Monocular Congenital Cataracts

Drummond GT, Scott WE, Keech RV (Univ of Iowa)
*Arch Ophthalmol* 107:45–51, January 1989

8–2

Fourteen patients with a diagnosis of monocular congenital cataract were seen from 1971 through 1985. All had a visually significant cataract at birth or before age 2 months. On follow-up, excellent distance linear recognition acuity correlated with earlier surgery, earlier contact lens fitting, and good compliance with amblyopia therapy. The oldest age for attainment of excellent or good visual acuity was 17 weeks. Patching began with 50% occlusion until age 2 months and then gradually increased to 100% after age 7 months. Six patients had a final visual acuity of better than 20/50 and 3 others had an acuity of 20/60 to 20/100 at follow-up.

The age at surgery and optical correction relates closely to the outcome in monocular congenital cataract. It is possible that deprivation amblyopia caused by such a cataract can be reversed as late as age 4 months in some instances. Compliance with an effective optical correction and patching program is important. Poor compliance either with wearing a contact lens or with patching compromises the visual outcome. The oldest age at which optical correction is consistent with good or excellent visual acuity remains unknown.

---

**Extended-Wear Contact Lenses for the Treatment of Pediatric Aphakia**
Levin AV, Edmonds SA, Nelson LB, Calhoun JH, Harley RD (Wills Eye Hosp, Philadelphia)
*Ophthalmology* 95:1107–1113, August 1988                                  8–3

---

One of the most common causes of blindness in children is cataracts. Early optical rehabilitation for pediatric aphakia is crucial to decrease the incidence of amblyopia, strabismus, and poor fusion. The advantages and disadvantages of the techniques used for refractive correction have been debated. The practicality of extended-wear contact lenses in the refractive correction of pediatric aphakia was evaluated in 184 patients with 240 affected eyes.

At the time of contact lens fitting, ages ranged from 18 days to 9.8 years. The 141 eyes fit from day 1 to 55 months after surgery were followed for 6 months to 5.7 years. Only 5 patients lost more than 5 lenses; the overall loss rate was less than 1 lens per year. None of the patients had contact lens–related complications with permanent visual consequences. Only 14% had contact lens problems or factors related to parental inability to care for the lens that resulted in discontinuation of use. No subset of patients who should be considered for primary surgical optical correction of aphakia could be identified.

Contact lens therapy is the optimal means of attempting primary rehabilitation in these patients. The procedure has a high success rate, low morbidity, and a wide range of applicability. A 100% silicone polymer extended-wear contact lens has been found most helpful.

▶ Optical correction of pediatric aphakia includes spectacles, contact lenses, intraocular lenses, and epikeratophakia. Extended-wear contact lenses are safe and effective in correcting pediatric aphakia. As the refractive error of the eye changes, the contact lenses can be modified appropriately. Extended-wear contact lenses should remain the primary means of correcting pediatric aphakia.—L.B. Nelson, M.D.

## Congenital and Traumatic Cataract: The Effect on Ocular Axial Length
Rasooly R, BenEzra D (Hadassah Univ Hosp, Jerusalem)
*Arch Ophthalmol* 106:1066–1068, August 1988                            8–4

Elongation of the eye is a drawback implanting intraocular lenses in children. The possible effects of cataract and aphakia on eye elongation were assessed in 42 children with unilateral aphakia and 22 with bilateral congenital cataract. Axial length was measured. The presumed rate of elongation was quantitatively expressed based on time elapsed since surgery and patient age.

In bilateral congenital cataract the axial length measured in surgically treated aphakic eyes was comparable to that in eyes not surgically treated. The significant association found between reduced visual acuity and increased axial length suggests a possible role of visual perception in modulating eye growth in infancy. However, the final ocular axial length is probably determined by other factors usually not readily detected. Excessive eye elongation may be associated with aphakia per se rather than with amblyopia or poor vision. However, in this series the mean axial length of bilateral aphakic eyes was not significantly different from that in bilateral phakic eyes.

Ocular dimensions may also be affected by changes in intraocular pressure or in tonus of the ciliary body. The multifactorial nature of eye growth may be the cause of the reported inconsistent association between amblyopia and eye elongation.

Unilateral cataract or aphakia appears to be associated with excessive eye elongation in affected eyes. Eye elongation seems to be related to amblyopia and poor vision rather than to aphakia.

▶ The correlation between eye elongation and amblyopia and poor vision rather than aphakia that the authors document is an important clinical finding. It is another possible argument against the use of intraocular lenses as a primary procedure to correct unilateral aphakia in infancy. However, the authors should have included the changes in actual refraction in their patients with unilateral and bilateral aphakia to make the study more clinically useful.—L.B. Nelson, M.D.

## The Nationwide Study of Epikeratophakia for Aphakia in Older Children
Morgan KS, McDonald MB, Hiles DA, Aquavella JV, Durrie DS, Hunkeler JD, Kaufman HE, Keates RH, Sanders DR (Louisiana State Univ; Univ of Pittsburgh; Univ of Rochester; Univ of Nebraska; Ohio State Univ; et al)
*Ophthalmology* 95:526–532, April 1988                            8–5

Epideratophakia alters the anterior curve of the cornea by adding a tissue lens shaped from the donor cornea. There are no cuts in the host cor-

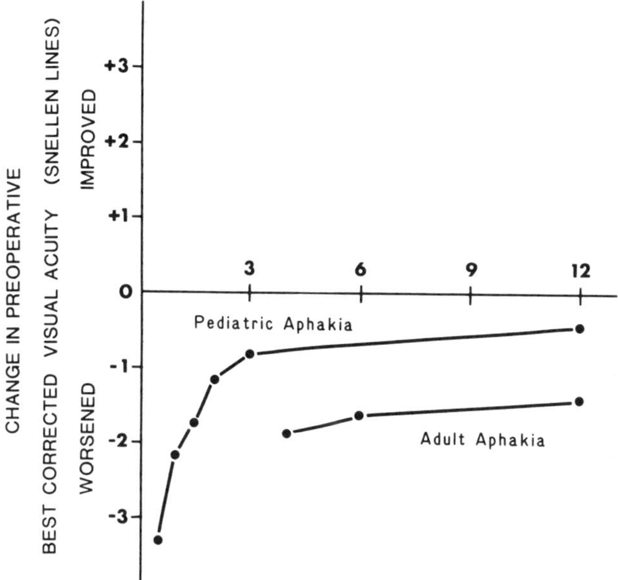


**Fig 8−2.**—Rate of recovery of vision in older children compared with aphakic adults. Recovery in children appears to be both more rapid and more complete than in older patients. *Horizontal axis* represents months after surgery. (Courtesy of Morgan KS, McDonald MB, Hiles DA, et al: *Ophthalmology* 95:526−532, April 1988.)

nea, and the recipient Bowman's layer is not damaged except for a 0.5-mm annular keratectomy. The procedure is extraocular, reversible, and adaptable to corneas of differing size and shape. The procedure is used to correct aphakia and myopia in adults and children, and to treat keratoconus.

Sixty-three patients aged 8−18 years underwent epikeratophakia in 65 eyes. Thirty-five patients had traumatic cataracts and 28 had congenital cataracts. Fifty-one eyes were aphakic at the time of surgery. All of the operations were successful. Seventy-three percent of patients were within 3 D of emmetropia postoperatively. Corrected acuity was somewhat more likely to improve in patients with congenital cataract than in those with traumatic cataract. Older children recovered vision better than adults did (Fig 8−2).

About three fourths of these children had correction within 3 D of emmetropia after epikeratophakia. Epikeratophakia is safer than intraocular lens implantation in older children with aphakia. The contact lens compliance rate for these patients is poor.

▶ The authors suggest that the risk-benefit ratio favors epikeratophakia over intraocular lenses in the pediatric age group. However, a controlled study is needed, performed by surgeons trained in both procedures, in which patients are randomly treated with either procedure. Visual acuity showed a slight tendency toward improvement in patients who underwent epikeratophakia after removal of a dense or incomplete cataract; a slight decrease in best corrected visual acuity was noted in traumatic cataract patients. Again, would intraocular lens insertion or continuation of contact lens or spectacle wear have altered the results?.—L.B. Nelson, M.D.

## Management of Traumatic Hyphema in Children: An Analysis of 340 Cases

Uusitalo RJ, Ranta-Kemppainen L, Tarkkanen A (Helsinki Univ)
*Arch Ophthalmol* 106:1207–1209, September 1988                    8–6

Various therapies have been used to treat traumatic hyphema. Studies were made in 340 children with nonperforating traumatic hyphema to verify or refute the possible protective action of the antifibrinolytic agent tranexamic acid against rebleeding.

In the first group studied retrospectively, traumatic hyphema in 219 children was treated with strict bed rest, binocular patching, and sedation but not antifibrinolytic agents. In the second group studied prospectively, 121 children received systemically administered tranexamic acid. Twenty-six children in the second group were confined to bed rest and 95 were allowed free ambulation in their rooms (table).

The frequency of secondary hemorrhage was 9.6% in the first group. Tranexamic acid reduced the incidence of secondary hemorrhage significantly: None of the 26 eyes in patients who received this agent and were confined to bed rest rebled, and only 1 (1.1%) of the 95 eyes in children who received the agent and were allowed ambulation rebled.

Tranexamic acid is effective in decreasing the incidence of secondary

Group Comparisons of Characteristics of Traumatic Hyphema in 340 Children*

| | Group 1 (n = 219) | Group 2 (n = 26) | Group 3 (n = 95) | P† |
|---|---|---|---|---|
| Age, y (mean ± SD) | 9.7 ± 3.3 | 10.8 ± 2.6 | 9.4 ± 3.1 | NS |
| % Male | 83.1 | 80.8 | 82.1 | NS |
| Hyphema grade, % | | | | |
| Grade 1 | 74.9 | 57.6 | 77.9 | NS |
| Grade 2 | 23.3 | 34.6 | 21.1 | NS |
| Grade 3 | 0.4 | 3.9 | 1.0 | NS |
| Grade 4 | 1.4 | 3.9 | 0.0 | NS |
| Resorption time of hyphema, d (mean ± SD) | 4.7 ± 2.6 | 5.6 ± 2.8 | 4.9 ± 2.8 | NS |
| No. (%) of rebleeding episodes | 21 (9.6) | 0 (0) | 1 (1.1) | <.01 |

*Group 1 was treated with bed rest only; group 2 with tranexamic acid and bed rest; and group 3 with tranexamic acid and patients were free to ambulate in their hospital room.
†The P value is derived from $\chi^2$ analysis between groups 1 and 3. NS, not significant.
(Courtesy of Uusitalo RJ, Ranta-Kemppainen L, Tarkkanen A: *Arch Ophthalmol* 106:1207–1209, September 1988.)

hemorrhage in children. The goal of treatment with this agent is to delay dissolution of the clot and to allow the proliferating cells to seal the gap in the traumatized vessels.

▶ Secondary hemorrhage in patients with traumatic hyphema is probably related to lysis and retraction of the clot and fibrin aggregates occluding the initially traumatized vessel. It certainly seems logical that an antifibrinolytic agent, such as tranexamic acid, would delay dissolution of the clot and prevent a secondary hemorrhage. An advantage of tranexamic acid over aminocaproic acid, another antifibrinolytic drug, is the lack of systemic side effects. I agree with the authors that the development of a topical antifibrinolytic agent would circumvent the problems of systemic side effects.

Also see Abstract 2–23 in this volume on aminocaproic acid.—L.B. Nelson, M.D.

---

**Errors in the Three-Step Test in the Diagnosis of Vertical Strabismus**
Kushner BJ (Univ of Wisconsin)
*Ophthalmology* 96:127–132, January 1989                                   8–7

---

Parks described a 3-step test for isolated cyclovertical muscle palsy based on the head-tilt phenomenon. However, other causes of vertical strabismus may incorrectly suggest a palsy of 1 cyclovertical muscle if this test is relied on. These include vertical rectus contracture, paresis of more than 1 vertical muscle, dissociated vertical divergence, previous vertical muscle surgery, myasthenia gravis, and small nonparalytic vertical deviations associated with horizontal strabismus.

Moore and Cohen found that patients with esotropia typically have elevations of each eye on contralateral tilting and depression on ipsilateral tilting. Exotropic patients typically have elevation on ipsilateral tilting and depression on contralateral tilting. Ocular rotations usually do not appear as substantial limitations or overactions, as occur with vertical muscle pareses. Also, in patients with oblique muscle palsy there tends to be a considerable difference in vertical deviation between right and left gaze.

In addition to the 3-step test, there should be testing for a secondary deviation, especially if acuity is unequal in the 2 eyes. Ocular rotations of both eyes should be assessed in the diagnostic fields of gaze, and qualitative cover testing should be done in the oblique fields of gaze. It is also necessary to know whether the hypertropia is of the dissociated type. A history of surgery is important. Skew deviation and myasthenia gravis are other important considerations.

---

**The Deterioration of Accommodative Esotropia: Frequency, Characteristics, and Predictive Factors**
Dickey CF, Scott WE (Univ of Iowa)
*J Pediatr Ophthalmol Strabismus* 25:172–175, July–August 1988          8–8

---

Accommodative esotropia initially controlled by spectacles may deteriorate in some patients. Factors accounting for deterioration were examined in a series of 114 patients with accommodative esotropia followed for at least 10 years.

In 15 patients (13%) deterioration was observed on follow-up. It was comparably frequent in the 73 patients with a normal accommodative convergence/accommodation (AC/A) ratio and in the 41 patients with a high ratio. Deterioration tended to be more frequent when there was a longer delay between the onset of esodeviation and the prescription of optical correction, and was most common when esodeviation began at or before age 2 years. Deterioration occurred in 21% of patients with moderate hyperopia and in 9% of those with a refractive error of +2.50 D or less.

Accommodative esotropia deteriorates relatively often in patients affected in the first 2 years of life. Patients with moderate hyperopia are those most likely to become worse. The AC/A ratio is not a predictive factor, but deterioration occurs more often, with a longer interval from the onset to hyperopic correction.

▶ The authors' findings should help the ophthalmologist to predict which children with acquired esotropia will not respond or may eventually have deterioration despite antiaccommodative therapy. The authors noted that deterioration occurred in statistically identical proportions of patients with normal and high AC/A ratios, which is contradictory to a recent article by Ludwig and co-workers (see Abstract 8–9) who found a greater deterioration rate in patients with a high AC/A ratio.—L.B. Nelson, M.D.

---

**Rate of Deterioration in Accommodative Esotropia Correlated to the AC/A Relationship**
Ludwig IH, Parks MM, Getson PR, Kammerman LA (Mary Imogene Bassett Hosp, Cooperstown, NY; George Washington Univ)
*J Pediatr Ophthalmol Strabismus* 25:8–12, January–February 1988          8–9

---

In some patients with accommodative esotropia a nonaccommodative component develops despite initial ocular alignment achieved with hypermetropic spectacles. The belief that the disorder deteriorates more often if the accommodation convergence (AC/A) relationship is high was examined in 119 patients whose eyes were aligned with spectacles alone. The AC/A relationships were graded according to the difference between near and distance measurements.

Thirty-six patients (30%) had deterioration, and it was more frequent in the high AC/A grades (table). With deterioration, a nonaccommodative component of esotropia of more than 10 at distance was superimposed on the initial accommodative esotropia. Deterioration was observed in 8% of patients with a normal AC/A and in 52% of those with a high AC/A of at least 30. Amblyopia was not significantly related to the outcome.

| | | AC/A Grade | | | |
|---|---|---|---|---|---|
| | Normal | Grade 1 | Grade 2 | Grade 3 | Total |
| Deteriorated | 3(7.9%)* | 6(25.0%) | 11(42.3%) | 16(51.6%) | 36(30.3%) |
| Undeteriorated | 35 | 18 | 15 | 15 | 83 |
| Total | 38 | 24 | 26 | 31 | 119 |

Deterioration by AC/A Grade

*Incidence of deterioration in parentheses.
$\chi^2 = 17.81$; $P < 0.001$.
(Courtesy of Ludwig IH, Parks MM, Getson PR, et al: *J Pediatr Ophthalmol Strabismus* 25:8–12, January–February 1988.)

Deterioration is most frequent in patients with accommodative esotropia who have a high AC/A relationship. Amblyopia was not a significant factor, but only mildly amblyopic patients were included in the study. It is possible that patients with a high AC/A relationship experience near esotropia repeatedly despite having bifocal spectacles and that, in time, the extraocular muscles are permanently damaged as a result.

▶ The rate of deterioration of accommodative esotropia after initial successful alignment with spectacles was greater in patients with a high AC/A relationship. Such patients may be experiencing near esotropia repeatedly, causing alterations in the structure of the extraocular muscles and leading to deteriorations.—L.B. Nelson, M.D.

## The Use of Vertical Offsets With Horizontal Strabismus Surgery

Metz HS (Univ of Rochester, NY)
*Ophthalmology* 95:1094–1097, August 1988                                  8–10

Operating on only the horizontal recti has the advantage of shortening the surgical time and leaving the vertical recti intact in patients with a vertical deviation coexisting with a large horizontal strabismus. However, concern has been expressed about the predictability of the results when displacing the horizontal rectus insertions vertically. A retrospective study was done to assess the efficacy of this approach.

Eighty-three patients had vertical displacement of the horizontal rectus muscle insertions monocularly along with recession-resection surgery to correct comitant vertical strabismus coexisting with a horizontal deviation. A surgical plan of about 1 mm of displacement of both the medial and lateral rectus insertions to correct each prism diopter of vertical deviation was used. Sixty-seven percent of patients had no residual vertical strabismus and 80% had vertical strabismus of no more than 2 prism diopters. The mean follow-up was 18 months. Little change was observed in the vertical deviation after the 1-month postoperative assessment. Transposition seemed to have no effect on the results of surgery for the horizontal strabismus.

There are several advantages to this operation. If a vertical rectus muscle is to undergo surgery for a comitant coexisting vertical strabismus, the opposite eye is usually selected for the vertical surgery, which avoids subjecting 3 adjacent rectus muscles to surgery and thus greatly diminishes the possibility of anterior segment ischemia, particularly in older patients. The surgeon who prefers to confine surgery to 1 eye because of amblyopia, however, cannot do this if a vertical rectus procedure on the other eye is elected. Vertically displacing the horizontal rectus insertions permits the surgery to be done on 1 eye. The time of surgery and anesthesia is reduced, and there is less postoperative reaction.

▶ Vertical displacement of the horizontal rectus muscles is an effective surgical procedure to correct comitant vertical strabismus coexisting with a horizontal deviation. This procedure is especially valuable when surgery must be performed on 1 eye, such as when amblyopia is present or retrobulbar anesthesia is used.—L.B. Nelson, M.D.

---

## Enhancing Surgery for Acquired Esotropia

Jotterand VH, Isenberg SJ (Univ of California, Los Angeles)
*Ophthalmic Surg* 19:263–266, April 1988                                     8–11

---

If only the nonaccommodative angle is operated on in acquired esotropia, undercorrection frequently results. An attempt was made to decrease the occurrence of such an outcome by enhancing surgery. A target angle equal to half the sum of the distant nonaccommodative angle [minimum, 12 prism diopters; (pd)] plus the distant angle measured without correction was sought. If, for example, a child had esotropia of 40 pd on distant fixation without correction and 20 pd with full hyperopic correction, the target angle was 30 pd. Either both medial recti were recessed or both lateral recti were resected.

Twenty operations were done on 18 patients. The mean esotropia on distant gaze was 45 pd without correction and 25 pd with correction. The mean augmentation was 0.8 mm in 12 patients having bimedial rectus recession and 1.7 mm in 8 patients having bilateral rectus resection after a previous bimedial rectus recession. Postoperatively, while wearing full hyperopic correction and fixating a distant target, the mean angle was 6 pd of esodeviation. Four patients were undercorrected. In 3 patients exotropia developed within 3 months of surgery while they were wearing their preoperative spectacles.

Patients with acquired esotropia that is only partly responsive to spectacle control of accommodation may benefit from enhanced surgery. The prism adaptation test may help to indicate which patients are likely to benefit. Overcorrected patients have become orthotropic after reduction of their hyperopic correction.

▶ Strabismus surgeons are often disappointed at the high rate of undercorrection after surgery for nonaccommodative esotropia. The authors discuss a unique mathematical formula for deriving the amount of medial rectus recession, but a larger series of patients with a control group using standard surgery is needed to verify their success.—L.B. Nelson, M.D.

## Bilateral Anterior Transposition of the Inferior Obliques

Mims JL III, Wood RC (Univ of Texas, San Antonio)
*Arch Ophthalmol* 107:41–44, January 1989
8–12

Sixty-one children with bilateral overaction of the inferior oblique muscle and previous or current infantile esotropia underwent bilateral inferior oblique recessions 2–4 mm anterior to the lateral end of the inferior rectus insertion (Fig 8–3). Anteriorization to more than 2 mm anterior to the lateral end of the rectus insertion was reserved for patients who also had significant dissociated vertical deviation.

One child later required surgery for dissociated vertical deviation and 1 required denervation and extirpation for recurrent overaction of an inferior oblique. The average follow-up was 27 months, and the average age at last visit was 62 months. Nine of 60 other patients with infantile esotropia who did not have inferior oblique surgery required operation for dissociated vertical deviation. Most of these patients had symmetric superior rectus recessions of 9–13 mm.

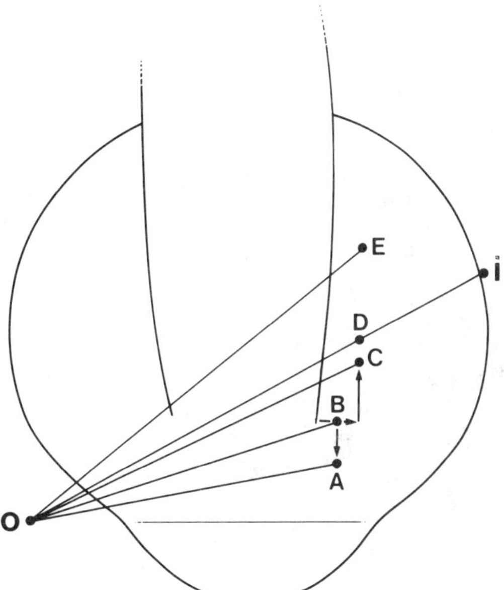


**Fig 8–3.**—Recession of inferior oblique to various points preferred by different surgeons. *Point A* is anterior transposition used in this study. *Point B* was favored by Elliott and Nankin. *Point C* is "10-mm" recession point of Parks. *Point D* was recommended by Apt and Call for moderate overaction of inferior oblique. *Point E* is "14-mm" recession point of Parks, favored by Hiles et al. Point i is insertion of inferior oblique and *point O* is insertion. (Courtesy of Mims JL III, Wood RC: *Arch Ophthalmol* 107:41–44, January 1989.)

Bilateral anterior transposition of the inferior oblique muscles effectively eliminates overaction of these muscles. Dissociated vertical deviation is reduced or prevented at the same time. The need for further surgery is considerably less than when inferior oblique surgery is not performed.

## Sequential Cranial Computed Tomography in Infants With Retinal Hemorrhages

Giangiacomo J, Khan JA, Levine C, Thompson VM (Univ of Missouri-Columbia)
*Ophthalmology* 95:295–299, March 1988                                    8–13

Unexplained retinal hemorrhages in infants that are not related to birth trauma or other significant trauma or disease should suggest cerebral trauma secondary to child abuse. Eisenbry suggested that such hemorrhages be taken as diagnostic of abuse in children younger than 3 years of age who lack external evidence of head injury.

Five whiplash-shaken infants who were lethargic and irritable, and had vomiting and intraocular bleeding, underwent cranial computed tomography (CT). In 3 of them there was a delay between intraocular and subdural hemorrhage. Recognition is easier after several days or weeks as cerebral edema declines and the subdural effusion enlarges. Brain atrophy may be accompanied by areas of massive infarction (Fig 8–4). Contrast-enhanced CT may help to identify thinner collections.

Unexplained retinal hemorrhages in an infant who has nonspecific signs of CNS irritability warrant continued monitoring of head circumference and the state of the optic disks, as well as repeat cranial CT as

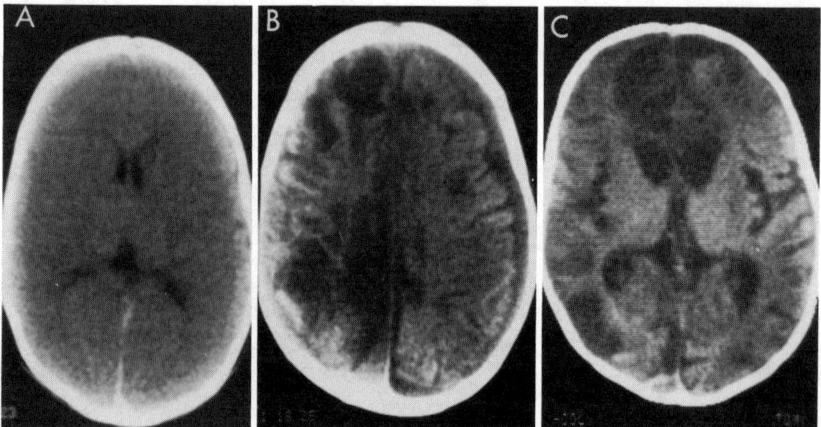

Fig 8–4.—**A,** the initial CT scan with contrast showing a small linear hyperdense area in the left frontal area *(arrowhead).* **B,** a CT scan 18 days later showing extensive cortical ischemic changes as well as a left subdural effusion *(arrowhead).* **C,** a CT scan after evaluation of the hematoma showing generalized decreased density consistent with multiple cerebral infarcts as well as a small left subdural hematoma *(arrowhead).* (Courtesy of Giangiacomo J, Khan JA, Levine C, et al: *Ophthalmology* 95:295–299, March 1988.)

clinically indicated. If retinal hemorrhages are not correlated with the subtle early CT findings of subdural hematoma, child abuse may be overlooked and the infant returned to a potentially lethal environment.

▶ Retinal hemorrhages in all children younger than 3 years of age without external evidence of head trauma should be considered diagnostic of child abuse until proven otherwise. The initial CT head scan may be normal or show subtle abnormalities that warrant continued monitoring of head circumference, optic nerves, and repeat head CT as clinically indicated.—L.B. Nelson, M.D.

# 9 Refractive Surgery

## Newer Techniques in Refractive Surgery

Juan J. Arentsen, M.D.
*Cornea Service, Wills Eye Hospital, Philadelphia, Pennsylvania*

Surgical and nonsurgical means of changing the curvature of the cornea have been at the forefront of interest for anterior segment surgeons. This interest has been fueled in the past 30 years by the pioneer work of Jose Barraquer in Columbia and, more recently, by Fjodorov in Russia. Both keratomileusis and radial keratotomy (as well as their spin-offs) are here to stay, in one way or another.

Parallel to the development of new techniques of refractive surgery, there have been changes in the expectations of surgeons and patients, the ways in which techniques and their results are being reported, and the economic aspects surrounding them, just to name a few.

Most techniques usually have been preceded by overenthusiasm, promises that are never fulfilled, and even sensationalism. Some of them have simply disappeared, as is the case with thermokertoplasty for keratoconus, which was being studied in the early 1970s (and thanks to which, through an NIH grant, I was able to finance my Cornea Fellowship). Others, after a great initial surge, have settled at a level well below what was originally expected; this is the case with radial keratotomy. I wonder how many millions of dollars were spent on pachymeters, diamond knives and other instruments, advertisements, courses, and the like, and how many surgeons today perform radial keratotomy on a regular basis.

A characteristic of these new technologies is their escalating price, to the point that they are already inaccessible to the majority of ophthalmologists in the United States. Further techniques to be discussed here will also be beyond the reach of many ophthalmology centers here and abroad. What is the point of developing yet unproven techniques that will benefit only the few?

Lasers in ophthalmology can be applied for different purposes because of the capability of their thermal effect (to produce burns), their optical breakdown (to section tissues), and, more recently, their capacity to produce photochemical reactions that result in the removal of tissue with minimal or no damage to adjacent tissues (1). The "excimer" laser ("excited dimmer") (the far ultraviolet line at 193 nm) is produced by charging the laser with argon and fluorine gases, which react together in a high-voltage field to produce an excited diatomic molecular species that is the active laser medium (2). Of the various gas combinations that emit the ultraviolet range, argon and fluorine gases with a wavelength of 193 seem to be the most effective and cause less tissue damage when cutting into the cornea.

Photoablation by the excimer laser produces a well-localized rupture of only those molecular bonds that have been irradiated by it. Theoretically, because the penetration of photons at this wavelength is less than 1 μm, surrounding tissues should not be affected (3). However, marked swelling of the stroma adjacent to cuts of up to 30% of normal thickness, as well as destruction of endothelial cells beneath the line of irradiation, have been reported (3). The endothelial cells would be affected by acoustic or shock waves rather than by direct laser photoablation.

Nevertheless, the excimer laser is capable of producing a clean and smooth cut, both in incisions (e.g., in radial keratotomy) and on full surfaces when "carving" a lamellar piece of cornea. On transmission electromicroscopy, corneas treated with excimer laser show "denatured" material on the surface that is 0.1−0.3 μm in thickness; beyond this damaged area the corneal structure seems to be normal (4).

The argon-fluorine laser operates with pulse energy densities of more than 400 mJ/sq cm at as many as 25 pulses per second. The area to be affected in the cornea is further delineated with the use of a mask in which the desired shape opening has been made, i.e., circular or slit-shaped. In terms of energy, 1 joule per sq cm ablates corneal tissue to a depth of 1 μm. In earlier reports a complete full-thickness section of the cornea took approximately 100 seconds to achieve (1). This was still much slower than a corneal cut with a diamond knife. The principal drawback with the excimer laser then was that it required different methods to fixate the globe (and the patient), e.g., local and general anesthesia (with all their dangers), headbands, and so on. Newer models of excimer lasers are capable of delivering higher amounts of energy in a shorter period of time and apparently allow the use of topical anesthesia (5). But other authors still believe that minor movements such as those induced by breathing or choroidal pulsation cannot be avoided and can affect the depth and shape of the incisions (6).

Further, the excimer laser can be used to cut plano corneal lenticules from fresh donor eyes, apparently at a much less cost than cryolathe-generated lenticules (7).

Unfortunately, newer developments in ophthalmology are always accompanied by quite undesirable situations; one is the press coverage of this work, such as a recent first-page article headed: "Prognosis for U.S. Excimer Patients, Good. First Operations Here Are Success," based on two procedures (one followed for 5 days and the other for an unspecified period of time) (8). According to the article, this study is being done under "FDA protocol;" if so, more discretion should be used before reporting any results. At the end of the article the editor comments that one of the surgeons in this FDA protocol has a proprietary interest in the company that manufactures that particular laser (!).

In yet another editorial regarding the ownership of a patent for the excimer laser used in corneal surgery, the editor speculates that if a patent were owned by an individual or company, other companies would be less enthusiastic about further research in the field of excimer lasers and corneal surgery (9). On the other hand, if a patent were held for the procedure, each time it was performed someone (e.g., surgeon, patient) would have to pay a license fee for its use. This would definitely stop progress in this area, and it is just an unthinkable suggestion (it reminds me of the Inquisition and certainly all dictatorships). Let's free the patents!

One aspect that has been at the core of all of the discussions in the field of refractive procedures (aside from safety and efficacy) has been predictability of the results. A few years ago an article in *Time* magazine, (written by an American) referred to two "loves" of the Americans: gadgets and predictability. According to this author, whose name escapes me now, Americans have a terrible urge to predict the future (in the market, sports, and weather, to name a few), to the point that major corporations used to have large staffs of economists whose only purpose was that of predicting. By the late '60s and '70s, when it was realized that predictions can be made only on a scientific basis (the rest being speculation), most of these economists were fired.

Something we have to realize is that no matter how precise and reproducible the effect of a knife or a laser or any other corneal cutting device may be, the cornea is not a static structure. The cornea is a living piece of tissue subject to constant changes, from external and internal pressures to metabolic and other interactions, many of them not well understood. These factors are much more important than the type of instrument that is used initially to modify the curvature and shape of the cornea. These procedures become popular and acceptable only when patients and surgeons understand that refractive surgery is and will always be unpredictable.

*References*

1. Shinivasan R, Braren B: "Excimer" laser surgery of the cornea. *Am J Ophthalmol* 96:710–715, 1983.
2. Krueger RR, Trokel SL, Schubert HD: Interaction of ultraviolet laser light with the cornea. *Invest Ophthalmol* 26:1455–1464, 1985.
3. Marshall J, Trokel S, Rothery S, et al: An ultrastructural study of corneal incisions induced by an excimer laser at 193 nm. *Ophthalmology* 92:749–758, 1985.
4. Puliafito CA, Steinert RF, Deutsch TF, et al: Excimer laser ablation of the cornea and lens. Experimental studies. *Ophthalmology* 92:741–748, 1985.
5. Schroder E, Dardenn MV, Neuhann T, et al: An ophthalmic excimer laser for corneal surgery. *Am J Ophthalmol* 103:472–473, 1987.
6. Aron-Rosa DS, Boerner CF, Bath P, et al: Corneal wound healing after excimer laser keratotomy in human eye. *Am J Ophthalmol* 103:454–464, 1987.
7. Gabay S, Slomovic A, Jares T: Excimer laser-processed donor corneal lenticules for lamellar keratoplasty. *Am J Ophthalmol* 107:47–51, 1989.
8. Bruch LB: Prognosis for U.S. excimer patients, good. First operations here are success. *Ophthalmol Times* 13:1, 26, 1988.
9. News Commentary: Patent fight erupts over excimer laser corneal surgery. *Refract Corneal Surg* 5:3, 1989.

## Surgical Correction of Postoperative Astigmatism

Lindstrom RL, Lindquist TD (Univ of Minnesota)
*Cornea* 7:138–148, 1988

9–1

The photokeratoscope has allowed more predictable models of surgical astigmatic correction. Factors in postoperative astigmatism include differential wound healing rates, irregular collagen deposition, and prolonged collagen remodeling.

Marked undercorrections and overcorrections have been achieved in postkeratoplasty astigmatism using relaxing incisions. Poor predictability is the chief problem with this procedure. Inadvertent perforation or wound dehiscence may occur when relaxing incisions are made. Careful dissection of the graft-host interface with a microsharp metal blade is necessary (Fig 9–1). More perforations occur when preset diamond knives are used. If incisions do not adequately correct astigmatism, compression sutures may be placed at about 75% depth to produce overcorrection of 33% to 50% (Fig 9–2).

Wedge resection is used to correct large degrees of postkeratoplasty astigmatism. Resection of 0.1 mm of tissue generally results in about 2 D of astigmatic correction. The flatter meridian is steepened about twice as much as the steeper one is flattened.

Wedge resection is done under retrobulbar anesthesia. A 90-degree or 3-clock-hour section of the keratoplasty wound is incised nearly to Descemet's membrane before the wedge of tissue is removed. Sutures are left for at least 8 weeks and then removed selectively.

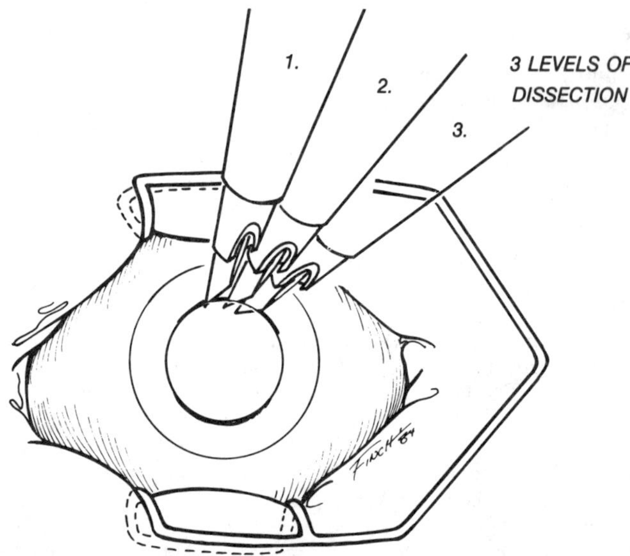


**Fig 9–1.**—Relaxing incision involves careful dissection of the graft-host interface for 90 degrees in a graded fashion. (Courtesy of Lindstrom RL, Lindquist TD: *Cornea* 7:138–148, 1988.)

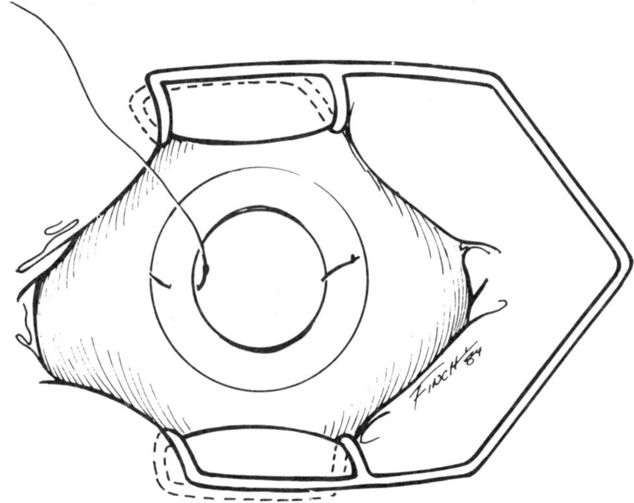

**Fig 9–2.**—Compression sutures are placed at 75% corneal depth on each side of the graft-host interface 90 degrees away from relaxing incisions. (Courtesy of Lindstrom RL, Lindquist TD: *Cornea* 7:138–148, 1988.)

Astigmatic keratotomy involves transverse or semiradial incisions, or a combination of these. In 124 cases a mean correction of 1.6 D resulted from a single pair of transverse incisions placed 5–8 mm apart. The closer the radial incisions are to the optical axis, the greater is the effect on corneal flattening. The maximum correction is achieved with a single set of transverse incisions placed 5 mm apart between 2 sets of semiradial incisions made from a 3-mm optical zone.

▶ Good guidelines are given on which procedure to use, depending on the degree of astigmatism resulting from keratoplasty. These are general rules and their results are still unpredictable in an important number of patients. No 2 surgeons perform a particular procedure in the same fashion.—J.J. Arentsen, M.D.

---

**Radial Keratotomy on Trial: New Surgical Procedures and the Antitrust Laws: Part 1**
Duffey WS Jr (King & Spalding, Atlanta)
*J Refract Surg* 4:232–239, November–December 1988                    9–2

Some surgeons in the United States wished to disseminate radial keratotomy without further study, whereas others believed that extensive investigation was in order. As a result a class action lawsuit was brought against physicians involved in the Prospective Evaluation of Radial Keratotomy (PERK) study and other groups on the grounds that they had conspired to restrain performance of radial keratotomy in volation of federal antitrust laws.

Two years later a similar suit was filed against the American Academy of Ophthalmology and its directors. Plaintiffs claimed to represent not only surgeons but also patients who wished to have this procedure and others who had had the operation and whose insurance carriers refused to pay. They contended that radial keratotomy was "branded" as an experimental procedure, but they did not attack the scientific grounds for the PERK study.

Defendants held that an "experimental" designation was appropriate so that physicians and the public would know that the efficacy and safety of the operation remained to be established. Defendants urged that it was reasonable to issue statements urging caution in performing the operation. Evidence was presented to show that thousands of radial keratotomy procedures had been done by ophthalmologists throughout the United States, indicating that there was no monopoly. A small minority of PERK surgeons have gone on to practice radial keratotomy extensively.

---

**Radial Keratotomy in the United States: The Turbulent Decade**
Waring GO (Atlanta)
*J Refract Surg* 4:204–208, November–December 1988                    9–3

---

Experience with radial keratotomy shows that properly designed clinical trials are the best way to determine the efficacy and safety of a new procedure. Conflict over such procedures is best resolved by vigorous debate among ophthalmologists and detailed reporting of clinical information, not by litigious actions and political manipulation.

Eager myopic patients responded to dramatic public reports on radial keratotomy, and the cautious majority of ophthalmologists feared that the procedure was being evaluated in the marketplace rather than in the clinic and laboratory. Powerful economic factors were involved. The struggle took place between enthusiastic innovators eager to promulgate radial keratotomy and traditional conservatives.

The Keratorefractive Society proposed that no single group of surgeons should exclusively evaluate a given procedure. The Society attempted unsuccessfully to get the American Academy of Ophthalmology (AAO) to view radial keratotomy more favorably. The Prospective Evaluation of Radial Keratotomy study ensued, and various groups of ophthalmologists became bogged down in rancorous debate regarding the merits of the procedure and the propriety of its widespread use.

By the late 1980s convincing data on radial keratotomy became available. At the same time, reduced insurance coverage dampened enthusiasm for the operation. Presently, about 10% of ophthalmologists in the United States routinely perform radial keratotomy, making it available to patients who wish to have it. The directors of the AAO have been absolved of having illegally conspired to restrain practice.

**Topographic Analysis and Visual Acuity After Radial Keratotomy**
McDonnell PJ, Garbus J, Lopez PF (Estelle Doheny Eye Inst, Los Angeles; Wilmer Ophthalmological Inst, Baltimore)
*Am J Ophthalmol* 106:692–695, December 1988                    9–4

Some patients have better uncorrected visual acuity after radial keratotomy than was expected from the change in spherical equivalent, as determined by cycloplegic refraction, and the change in corneal curvature, as determined by keratometry. The topographic aspects of radial keratotomy were examined in 11 eyes of 6 patients using the Corneal Modeling System, a method of computed topographic analysis. With this method illuminated rings are reflected by the cornea and projected by a digital video system. The ring images are digitized and curves are fit to describe the shape of the entire corneal surface. The data are then translated into a color-coded topographic map.

In this study all of the eyes had fairly round zones of corneal flattening roughly centered around the corneal apex. These zones averaged 6.2 mm in diameter. In 3 eyes with markedly improved acuity despite substantial residual refractive errors, zones of relatively greater flattening were present within the larger circular area of flattening. A more uniform zone of flattening was present in eyes in which good acuity correlated with a nearly complete reduction in refractive error.

Patients with residual myopic refractive error after radial keratotomy may have better acuity than unoperated-on persons with a similar refractive error. The topographic changes in these patients may be analogous to concentric bifocal contact lenses. Further topographic studies may make it possible to intervene surgically in eyes with undesired optical zone changes to achieve a single relatively large optical zone and improve the quality of the retinal image.

---

**Two-Year Results of Reoperations for Radial Keratotomy**
Sawelson H, Marks RG (Cedars Med Ctr, Miami; Univ of Florida, Gainesville)
*Arch Ophthalmol* 106:497–501, April 1988                    9–5

The 2-year results of 320 radial keratotomy procedures not followed by reoperation were compared with those in 67 patients who were reoperated on. Follow-up was possible in 76% of the patients operated on once and in 79% of those reoperated on. Reoperation generally was planned at least 6 months after initial surgery. If 8 incisions were planned for both procedures, the later ones were made between the existing incisions. The optical zone size was chosen by treating the eye as a virgin case and therefore could differ from that in the first operation.

Eyes reoperated on averaged 2.2 D more initial myopia than those not having reoperation. The average myopia correction initially was 43% in the reoperated-on eyes and 84% in the others. Reoperation corrected an additional 47% of residual myopia for an overall correction of 70%.

Eyes having repeat radial keratotomy tend to be those of younger patients with greater initial myopia. The present findings suggest that twice the desired effect of correction should be attempted in a reoperation to achieve the desired outcome. Rather than treating reoperations as virgin cases, surgeons select the surgical parameters that predict the desired outcome.

▶ This study illustrates the well-known fact that the same amount of surgery has far less effect in reoperations than in primary radial keratotomy.—J.J. Arentsen, M.D.

---

**Irregular Astigmatism After Radial and Astigmatic Keratotomy**
McDonnell PJ, Caroline PJ, Salz J (Univ of Southern California, Los Angeles)
*Am J Ophthalmol* 107:42–46, January 1989                              9–6

---

Combined radial keratotomy and astigmatic keratotomy can produce complications, including irregular astigmatism when the incisions intersect. In 11 eyes (6 patients) intersecting radial and transverse corneal incisions led to substantial irregular corneal astigmatism. In all 6 patients planned intersecting incisions were made at the same time as the radial incisions. Four different surgeons had operated on these patients.

Best corrected acuity decreased in all eyes, and only 5 of the 11 eyes had vision of 20/40 or better with spectacles. Contact lenses were superior to spectacles in all instances; all eyes but 1 achieved acuity of 20/40 or better. Most eyes were succesfully fitted with rigid gas-permeable contact lenses. Slit-lamp study showed separation of the incision edges where the incisions intersected, with the gaps filled by epithelial plugs that extended down into the incisions. Photokeratoscopy showed moderate to marked irregular astigmatism, chiefly localized to the meridians with intersecting incisions.

Some irregular astigmatism may occur with radial incisions alone. If transverse incisions are added but do not intersect with the radial ones, the corneal contour remains fairly regular. If the topography is very irregular, however, contact lenses may be difficult to fit. Penetrating keratoplasty is an option in these cases. Alternatively, an attempt may be made to remove the epithelial plugs from sites of incisional crossing and then resuture the incisions. Surgeons should reconsider the practice of purposefully crossing incisions.

---

**Ruptured Globe Secondary to Blunt Trauma Following Radial Keratotomy**
Simons KB, Linsalata RP, Zaragosa AM (Univ of Arizona; Jules Stein Eye Inst, Los Angeles)
*J Refract Surg* 4:132–135, July–August 1988                              9–7

Because deep corneal incisions are recommended in radial keratotomy, several authors have been concerned about the risk of rupture of the corneal wounds after blunt trauma to the eye. The ocular integrity subsequent to radial keratotomy has been less than that of unoperated-on eyes in animals and in cadaver eyes. A patient was seen after he sustained a ruptured globe secondary to blunt trauma 24 days after radial keratotomy.

Man, 43, underwent a 4-incision radial keratotomy in the left eye. Before the procedure the best visual acuity was 2/70 OU without correction. After surgery, acuity was 20/40 without correction. The patient was later struck in the eye by an elbow and the globe ruptured. The eye was repaired primarily but enucleated subsequently. Histologic examination by light microscopy revealed a sutured, full-thickness corneal perforation. A radial keratotomy incision was observed adjacent to the perforation. Bowman's membrane was disrupted, and a hypercellular scar extending to two thirds the depth of the corneal stroma was noted. Descemet's membrane was intact under this incision site.

The findings demonstrate that eye integrity after radial keratotomy can be compromised. Two of the 4 radial keratotomy incisions were intact; however, the other 2 were not identified because of the severely deformed globe. The most extensive portion of the globe's rupture was within the cornea. At the very least, patients undergoing radial keratotomy should be advised of potential complications from blunt trauma and to use protective eyewear.

▶ We agree with the recommendations of the author that after radial keratotomy patients should wear protective glasses in any potentially dangerous situation. This applies to any instance in which the cornea has been cut, whether traumatically or surgically.—J.J. Arentsen, M.D.

---

## Hexagonal Keratotomy in Human Cadaver Eyes

Gilbert ML, Friedlander M, Aiello JP, Granet N (Tulane Univ)
*J Refract Surg* 4:12–14, January–February 1988                    9–8

---

Hexagonal keratotomy was carried out on 9 phakic human cadaver eyes unsuitable for corneal transplantation, without past surgery or disease, to estimate the keratometric and photokeratoscopic changes. A 5-mm central hexagonal keratotomy was done using the operating biomicroscope to an estimated 85% corneal depth. A 10.30-D increase in keratometric power resulted. Photokeratoscopy showed central corneal steepening compared with the naive eye, and computer analysis confirmed a significant increase in central steepness.

Hexagonal keratotomy has been proposed for the treatment of mild hyperopia. Visual distortion may result, but the present findings suggest that it is within acceptable limits. Predictable results depend on consistent incisions, precise pachymetry, and good blade depth measurements. The refractive effect is expected to vary with the size of the optical zone and the incision depth.

▶ Hexagonal keratotomy is in its very preliminary stages. Some of its promoters in foreign countries have abandoned it. Further experimental studies are mandatory.—J.J. Arentsen, M.D.

## Hexagonal Keratotomy for Corneal Steepening

Grady FJ (Univ of Texas, Houston)
*Ophthalmic Surg* 19:622–623, September 1988                              9–9

Radial keratotomy, introduced almost a decade ago, has received mixed acceptance by the ophthalmologic community. One criticism of the procedure is its imprecision. During the past 3 years Mendez has performed nearly 200 hexagonal keratotomies for hyperopia with excellent results. Hexagonal keratotomy was assessed for treatment of hyperopia, presbyopia, and radial keratotomy overresponse.

Data on 16 patients were reviewed. Five had radial keratotomy overcorrection, 5 had hyperopia, and 6 had presbyopia. The amount of correction desired was 1–4 D in all cases. With the optical zone marked as much as it would be for radial keratotomy, a Mendez hexagonal marker was placed on the cornea symmetrically around the pupil and each of the 6 sides was cut with a front-cutting Micra double-edged diamond at a depth of 80% of the central corneal pachymetry. After the hexagon was completely cut, each side was checked to ensure that it progressed completely into the adjacent incision, so that there were no areas of incomplete cut.

A monocular dressing, applied over NeoDecadron drops, was removed the next morning. A significant effect was evident on the first preoperative day, as with radial keratotomy. However, the overcorrection was not as large as with radial keratotomy and the regression was, at most, 1 D.

Hexagonal keratotomy appears to be a reasonably successful treatment of radial keratotomy overcorrection from excessive surgery or patient overresponse to the procedure. It also seems to be useful for treating low hyperopia and some presbyopia. Although hexagonal keratotomy is technically much more difficult than radial keratotomy, only time will tell if this therapy merits a permanent place in the armamentarium of ophthalmic refractive surgery.

▶ Results of hexagonal keratotomy for corneal steepening in only 16 of 200 patients are just not enough. Much more investigation of this technique, and certainly the results in the other 184 patients, is necessary before any conclusions or recommendations can be made.—J.J. Arentsen, M.D.

**Paired Arcuate Keratotomy: A Surgical Approach to Mixed and Myopic Astigmatism**
Duffey RJ, Jain VN, Tchah H, Hofmann RF, Lindstrom RL (Univ of Minnesota)
*Arch Ophthalmol* 106:1130–1135, August 1988                    9–10

Many surgical procedures have been advocated for correcting severe corneal astigmatism, including wedge resection, relaxing incision, relaxing incision with augmentation sutures, transverse incision, and trapezoidal astigmatic keratotomy. Arcuate or relaxing incisions are curved incisions that parallel the limbus; the length of each incision is equidistant from the center of the cornea. The degree of astigmatism induced by paired arcuate relaxing incisions was quantified in 25 cadaver eyes with minimal or no preoperative astigmatism.

Paired arcuate incisions placed at optical zones of 5, 6, 7, 8, and 9 mm were lengthened progressively from 45 to 60, 90 and 120 degrees. The corneal flattening in the meridian centered over the incisions and the corneal steepening 90 degrees away were quantified with each lengthening.

Linear regression analysis revealed a direct linear relationship of corneal astigmatic change to decreasing optical zone measured in millimeters and increasing incision length measured in degrees. The $\Delta K$ value ranged from a mean of 2.65 D to 22.05 D; the flattening/steepening coupling ratio mean was 1.47 (Fig 9–3).

Progressively longer paired arcuate incisions produced predictable and titratable corneal flattening in the meridian centered over the incisions

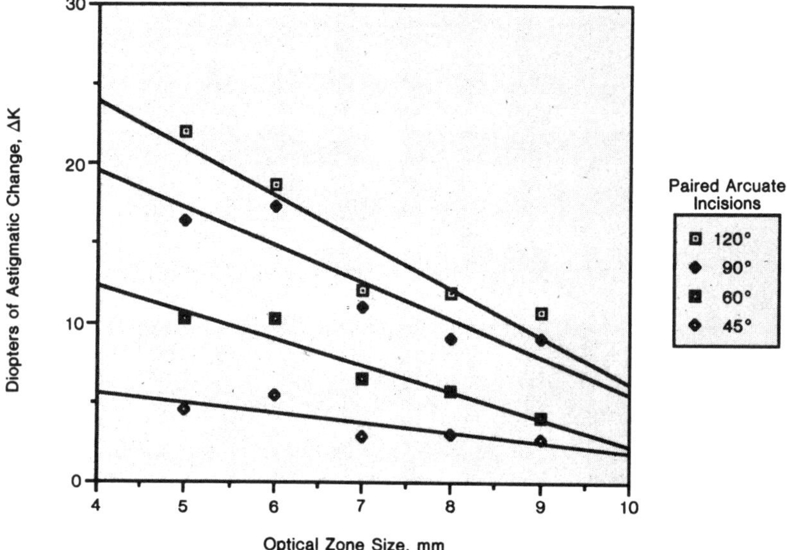


Fig 9–3.—Superimposed regression lines demonstrating linear relationship of sum of corneal flattening and steepening ($\Delta K$) to optical zone size for paired arcuate incisions of 45, 60, 90 and 120 degrees at optical zones of 5 through 9 mm. (Courtesy of Duffey RJ, Jain VN, Tchah H, et al: *Arch Ophthalmol* 106:1130–1135, August 1988.)

and slightly less corneal steepening 90 degrees away. This makes the procedure ideal for treating mixed astigmatism.

▶ Relaxing incisions have produced relatively good (although unpredictable) results in correcting slight astigmatism. The question remains, can results from cadaver eyes be transposed to living tissue, which is subject to constant change?—J.J. Arentsen, M.D.

**Clinical Results and Complications of Trapezoidal Keratotomy**
Villaseñor RA, Stimac GR (North Valley Eye Med Group, Inc, Mission Hills, Calif)
*J Refract Surg* 4:125–131, July–August 1988                    9–11

Trapezoidal keratotomy, or the Ruiz procedure, consisted initially of 2 semiradial plus 5 equally spaced transverse incisions on each side of the steepest corneal axis. The incision depth was varied from 40% to 80% of the pachymetry reading over the selected optic zone. Ruiz subsequently developed a nomogram that predicted the required optic zone and incision depth needed to correct various degrees of astigmatism. Trapezoidal keratotomy was done on 35 eyes using the various Ruiz nomograms and computer programs.

*Technique.*—Usually, the surgical technique was standard. A double-edged diamond knife was set at 100% of central pachymetry for optic zones of 4 mm or more. Incisions were made in a front cutting manner. The visual axis was marked with a blunt 30-gauge needle, using the corneal reflex from the microscope. A surgical keratometer was not used. The optic zone was marked, followed by transverse epithelial indentations 4 mm long using the Moria rake; semiradial indentations were not made. Transverse incisions on either side of the optic zone were placed first, after the indentations. When the trapezoidal and semiradial incisions were completed on 1 side, the first transverse incision made on the opposite side at the optic zone resulted in a high incidence of microperforations. The procedure was modified so that the 2 transverse incisions were placed at the optic zone first.

Clinical results in patients with postkeratoplasty astigmatism were significantly worse than in patients with congenital astigmatism. In 29 patients the astigmatism was actually increased. A greater lack of predictability was observed in this group than in any of the others. In patients with congenital astigmatism the degree of astigmatism was reduced in all but 1 patient. There was considerable lack of predictability in eyes with similar optic zones. The complication rate was high. Microperforations and macroperforations, large postoperative axis shifts, glare, spontaneous wound separation, and vascularization of the incisions were noted.

In this series, the results of trapezoidal keratotomy were unpredictable, especially in patients with postkeratoplasty astigmatism. Wound revisions and modifications of trapezoidal keratotomy were suggested for correction of large astigmatic refractive errors.

▶ This series on the Ruiz procedure probably reports the highest incidence of complications ever published. Once again, different refractive techniques have different results in different hands.—J.J. Arentsen, M.D.

## Long-Term Comparison of Epikeratoplasty and Penetrating Keratoplasty for Keratoconus

Steinert RF, Wagoner MD (Massachusetts Eye and Ear Infirmary, Boston; Harvard Med School)
*Arch Ophthalmol* 106:493–496, April 1988                     9–12

The results of epikeratoplasty for keratoconus in 10 patients followed for a mean of 25 months were compared with the outcome in 10 others having penetrating keratoplasty and followed for 33 months. The mean preoperative visual acuity was slightly worse for the patients having penetrating keratoplasty and the cones were steeper. The selection process for epikeratoplasty was biased toward patients having less steep, clear cones.

The mean postoperative spectacle acuity was 20/29 in the epikeratoplasty group after excluding a patient with 20/200 acuity who went on to penetrating keratoplasty. Spectacle acuity, refraction, and keratometric findings were similar in the 2 groups. The time of healing to best corrected acuity averaged 12 months in the epikeratoplasty group and 3 months in those having penetrating keratoplasty.

Only the time to recovery of stable visual acuity differed significantly in these operative groups. Penetrating keratoplasty would be preferable if rapid recovery of good acuity is important, as in a patient with occupational impairment because of advanced bilateral keratoconus. Otherwise, epikeratoplasty avoids intraocular surgical hazards and immune rejection, as well as permanent weakening of the globe and the associated risk of wound dehiscence. Refinements in topographic analysis may allow better selection of patients for epikeratoplasty.

▶ The authors with 2 dissimilar groups of patients show that, at present, epikeratoplasty has no significant advantages over keratoplasty in the treatment of keratoconus. Keratoplasty continues to be the surgical modality of choice in keratoconus.—J.J. Arentsen, M.D.

## Postoperative Management of Epikeratoplasty

Steinert RF, Grene RB (Harvard Med School; Univ of Kansas, Wichita)
*J Cataract Refract Surg* 14:255–264, May 1988                     9–13

Restoration of an intact epithelium is essential in the first 2 weeks after epikeratoplasty when devitalized human corneal tissue is implanted onto

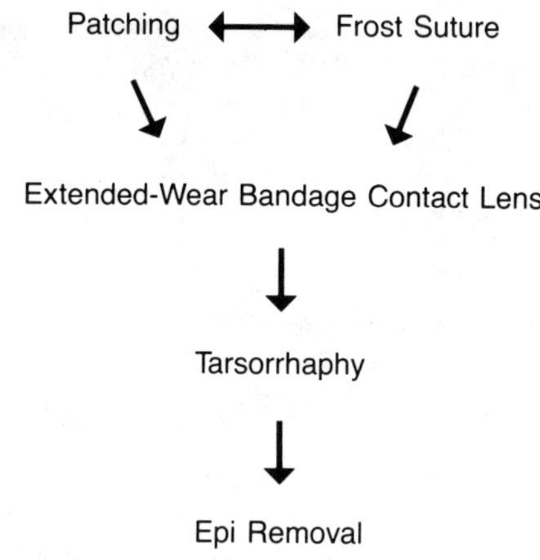



**Fig 9–4.**—Schematic approach to treatment alternatives for persistent epithelial defects. (Courtesy of Steinert RF, Grene RB: *J Cataract Refract Surg* 14:255–264, May 1988.)

a cornea for optical rehabilitation. On average, reepithelialization should be established within a week of surgery, and there should be 50% reepithelialization by day 4. Most physicians prefer to use an extended-wear bandage soft contact lens, a pressure patch, temporary central tarsorrhaphy, or an upper lid suture taped to the cheek. If reepithelialization is delayed, a patch or tarsorrhaphy is indicated (Fig 9–4).

Sterile infiltrates on nylon sutures are frequent after restoration of the epithelium, particularly in the inflamed eye with a localized ciliary flush. However, frank bacterial infiltration is infrequent. Loose sutures should be removed immediately, and tight sutures removed selectively to minimize astigmatism. Corneal edema is most common in aphakic eyes of elderly patients. The intraocular pressure should be determined. If edema persists, sodium chloride eyedrops and ointment may be effective, as well as steroids. Penetrating keratoplasty may be necessary if a borderline endothelium decompensates.

After full suture removal the emphasis is on visual rehabilitation. A year or more may be required for stable best-corrected spectacle acuity, especially in an older aphakic patient or a patient with keratoconus. Hard contact lenses are used when appropriate if irregular astigmatism is present. Decreased lens clarity may reflect delayed epithelialization, persistent edema, or scarring.

▶ The final results in eyes after epikeratoplasty depend not only on good preoperative evaluation (and indications) but, as importantly, on meticulous follow-up for a prolonged period of time.—J.J. Arentsen, M.D.

---

**The Surgical Management of Overcorrection in Myopic Epikeratophakia**
Nichols BD, Lindstrom RL, Spigelman AV (Univ of Minnesota)
*Am J Ophthalmol* 105:354–356, April 1988                                              9–14

Overcorrection resulted in 3 patients having epikeratophakia for myopia. It was confirmed after suture removal, a mean of 6 months postoperatively. Surgery for overcorrection was performed as an outpatient procedure under retrobulbar and facial nerve block anesthesia. After irrigation to remove epithelial debris, the trephination groove and peripheral corneal lamellar dissection plane were fractured open anterior to the wing of the lenticule using a Sinsky hook. Eight interrupted 10–0 nylon sutures then were placed through the wing of the lenticule using a slip-knot technique. Tension was adjusted to optimize corneal steepening; the best amount was at least equal to the degree of overcorrection.

The average postepikeratophakia spherical equivalent was +5.62 D. Uncorrected acuity ranged from 20/60 to 20/400. Best-corrected acuity generally was unchanged after resuturing, but uncorrected acuity improved dramatically in all 3 patients. The average spherical equivalent 2.8 months after the procedure was +0.75 D.

There is considerable variability in the refractive results of myopic epikeratophakia because the lenticule relies on the shoulder of the button to effect its minus power, and this is where suturing takes place. If overcorrection occurs, resuturing of the myopic lenticule to flatten the peripheral curvature can lessen the induced hyperopia.

▶ This article reminds us, again, that candidates for refractive surgery in general should very well understand what to expect before surgery.—J.J. Arentsen, M.D.

---

## Complications of Epikeratophakia

Grabner G (Univ of Vienna)
*J Refract Surg* 4:96–104, May–June 1988

9–15

---

Epikeratophakia is a reasonably reversible and repeatable treatment for aphakia, myopia, and keratoconus. A review was made of the current literature and data on 105 personal cases treated in a 3-year period. The excessive use of alcohol to remove the epithelium may cause corneal clouding and require penetrating keratoplasty. Surgical results are greatly improved by using cocaine or a blunt spatula, or both, and by careful attention to the peripheral epithelial ring. Incomplete removal of epithelium can lead to epithelial ingrowth or interface cysts. Perforation may result from incorrect use of the trephine or too deep an annular keratectomy. Shallow trephination can lead to problems when peripheral undermining is done with the Suarez spreader.

Early postoperative corneal complications are more frequent in epikeratophakia than with other lamellar procedures. Close follow-up is necessary to ensure early, complete reepithelialization. If epithelialization fails, central scarring or melting of the stromal cap may result. Filamentary keratitis sometimes is seen in myopic patients.

Persistent paracentral epithelial defects developed in 3 of 15 patients with keratoconus. Wound dehiscence occurred in 4 of these patients, making resuturing or replacement of the lenticule necessary.

Wrinkling of Bowman's layer and the stromal fold may lead to removal of apparently oversized lenticules. One patient had endothelial decompensation in Fuch's corneal endothelial dystrophy 3 years after successful epikeratophakia. Long-term studies of endothelial cell density in aphakic patients are needed.

A patient who had high myopia and retinal detachment caused by a hole at the posterior pole underwent successful repair. In another patient, progressive myopic macular changes lowered acuity substantially. Two patients with steroid glaucoma responded to withdrawal of treatment. Cystoid macular edema has been described in aphakic patients.

▶ In this author's experience, the incidence of complications in 105 patients with epikeratophakia seems quite high compared to that associated with alternative methods to correct ametropia.—J.J. Arentsen, M.D.

---

**Excimer Laser Radial Keratotomy in the Living Human Eye: A Preliminary Report**
Tenner A, Neuhann T, Schroder E, Salz JJ, Maguen E (Wangen, West Germany; Munich; Heroldsberg, West Germany; Cedars-Sinai Med Ctr, Los Angeles)
*J Refract Surg* 4:5–8, January–February 1988                    9–16

---

Radial keratotomy was performed using the Meditec excimer laser on the blind eyes of 3 volunteers. The argon fluoride excimer laser emits at a wavelength of 193 nm. A slit mask was developed to control the dimensions of the beam when it is projected onto the cornea. Peribulbar bupivacaine anesthesia and topical anesthesia with Pontocaine were used.

Eight radial incisions were made at about 50% to 60% of the corneal thickness with a 5.0-mm optical zone, resulting in 1–2 D of corneal flattening. The incisions were difficult to visualize and appeared nearly translucent; they regularly produced a fine double contour, probably because the laser excises corneal tissue rather than incising it.

Excimer laser radial keratotomy is a safe procedure in the living human eye. Eventually, this method may provide for more accurate incision depth and therefore more accurate refractive results. The laser incisions/excisions appear to produce less visible scars than conventional methods do. Excimer laser keratotomy reduces the refractive power of the cornea by corneal flattening. The degree of flattening is at least as great as with conventional keratotomy using an equal optical zone diameter, incision depth, and number of cuts.

▶ This preliminary study demonstrates that excimer laser radial keratotomy, although a promising technique, is still experimental and in its very early stages.—J.J. Arentsen, M.D.

## Human Excimer Laser Keratectomy: Short-Term Histopathology

L'Esperance FA Jr, Taylor DM, Warner JW (Columbia Univ; Univ of Connecticut, Farmington; Taunton Technologies, Inc, Monroe, Conn)
*J Refract Surg* 4:118–124, July–August 1988                    9–17

Reports that ultraviolet radiation emitted by excimer lasers can be used to etch submicron-sized patterns into the surface of plastics and other polymers with remarkable accuracy and no degradation of nearby unirradiated areas prompted research of the incisional and overall photoetching capabilities of far ultraviolet laser spectral emissions to establish a reconstructive superficial keratectomy or a new refractive curvature on the anterior surface of the cornea. Three human eyes were treated with argon fluoride excimer laser irradiation to produce a controlled superficial lamellar keratectomy.

*Technique.*—The Questek Model 1020 TOPS excimer laser combined with a delivery system was used. The eyes were stabilized with a vacuum ring that gently holds the eye in an upright position while the patient is supine. Globe fixation is maintained for only several minutes, but the laser's optics and the eye must be perfectly aligned throughout the procedure. Anesthesia of the cornea and anesthesia and akinesia of extraocular muscles were produced by retrobulbar or peribulbar injection of 2% lidocaine. After stabilization of the eye, the epithelium was removed. Photoablation was begun at a repetition rate of about 10 Hz and with a pulsed energy density (fluence) of 80–125 mJ/sq cm at the cornea. The procedure requires 35–45 seconds to create, from the surface of Bowman's membrane into the anterior stroma of the eye, an ablation to a depth of 30–40 μ.

In less than 14 days all three eyes reepithelialized completely, showing absolute clarity of all layers of the cornea. Patients had minimal discomfort. Histopathologic analysis showed the epithelium to be slightly hyperplastic but firmly adherent to the underlying stromal fibers in the ablated areas. A slight electron-dense border was seen at the epitheliostromal interface, but there was no evidence of inflammation or abnormal keratocyte activity.

Laser superficial keratectomy is a promising surgical intervention for reconstructive or refractive keratoplasty. Intensive investigations are needed of the corneal wound healing process after laser ablation and the nature and long-term stability of the corneal excisions or induced refractive corrections.

▶ Excimer keratectomy still needs further simplification and refinement in its initial stages before we even think that it will ever become a practical approach to changing the refractive power of the cornea.—J.J. Arentsen, M.D.

## Pseudophakic Bullous Keratopathy

Cohen EJ, Brady SE, Leavitt K, Lugo M, Speaker MG, Laibson PR, Arentsen JJ (Wills Eye Hosp, Philadelphia)
*Am J Ophthalmol* 106:264–269, September 1988                    9–18

The records of all outpatients with pseudophakic bullous keratopathy seen in a 6-month study period were reviewed to determine predisposing factors, associated problems, current management, and visual outcome. The study comprised 271 eyes in 251 patients aged 58–93 years, some of whom were seen for the first time and some of whom were seen in follow-up. Data were also collected regarding patients who had undergone penetrating keratoplasty.

Pseudophakic bullous keratopathy was associated with anterior chamber intraocular lenses in 155 of 271 eyes and with Leiske-style lenses in particular in 100 of these 271 eyes. At the initial examination pseudophakic bullous keratopathy was associated with visual acuity of 20/200 or less in 206 eyes and of counting fingers or less in 129 eyes.

Penetrating keratoplasty was performed in 189 eyes. After postoperative follow-up of 12–23 months, 108 of the treated eyes had visual acuity of 20/200 or less, but visual acuity improved with longer follow-up. Among patients with a minimum follow-up of 2 years, 23 of 36 eyes had visual acuity of 20/100 or better. Pseudophakic bullous keratopathy was associated with marked visual loss, which was permanent despite clear grafts in 29 of 92 eyes followed for 1 year or longer.

When the fate of the intraocular lens was correlated with the type used and the year of operation, it was found that 23 of 25 posterior chamber lenses were left in place, 21 of 58 iris-fixated lenses were left in place, and 26 were exchanged; 56 of 93 anterior chamber lenses were left in place and 27 were exchanged. The exchanged intraocular lenses were all replaced by an open-loop Kelman Multiflex anterior chamber lens.

Pseudophakic bullous keratopathy is clearly a common problem. In this series the differences between time of onset of corneal decompensation after implantation of various intraocular lenses had significant implications related to the types of lenses used. Preexisting endothelial dystrophy predisposed to early corneal decompensation in some patients undergoing extracapsular cataract extraction and posterior lens implantation. Although prolonged follow-up after corneal transplantation is always recommended, it is particularly important in patients with pseudophakic bullous keratopathy.

▶ The Leiske-style anterior chamber lens continues to be responsible for most pseudophakic bullous keratopathy developing after cataract extraction with intraocular lens implantation. This lens should always be exchanged or removed with keratoplasty for pseudophakic bullous keratopathy. Although most grafts remain clear after keratoplasty for pseudophakic bullous keratopathy, the visual acuity results are not nearly as good. There was marked visual loss in about one third of the patients with clear grafts followed for 1 year or longer in this study.—P.R. Laibson, M.D.

---

## Long-Term Healing of the Central Cornea After Photorefractive Keratectomy Using an Excimer Laser

Marshall J, Trokel SL, Rothery S, Krueger RR (Univ of London; Columbia-Presbyterian Med Ctr, New York)
*Ophthalmology* 95:1411–1421, October 1988                                    9–19

If submicron control of tissue removal by excimer laser radiation is possible by photorefractive keratectomy, it should be possible to ablate the equivalent of a contact lens onto the corneal surface. An excimer laser at 193 nm was used to ablate disks 3 mm in diameter from monkey corneas at varying depths up to 130 μm. Microscopy was carried out within 4–5 weeks and 6–8 months postoperatively.

Except with the deepest ablation, the corneas were clear immediately after operation. At 1 month ablations of 40 μm remained clear. Disks cut at 60 μm were clear at 6 months. Haze persisted on slit-lamp examination in the deepest disks. Reepithelialization occurred within 48 hours of the procedure. Stromal vacuolation had nearly resolved by 6 months, when keratocyte numbers were nearly normal. Morphological features were nearly normal by 8 months except for the absence of Bowman's membrane and some disorganization of the immediate subepithelial stroma.

Precise ablation of corneal tissue by photorefractive keratectomy (Fig 9–5) holds promise for clinical use. Corneal scatter remains but has not caused significant visual dysfunction. Pulsed laser delivery limits the risk of damaging adjacent tissues. The pseudomembrane that forms helps to

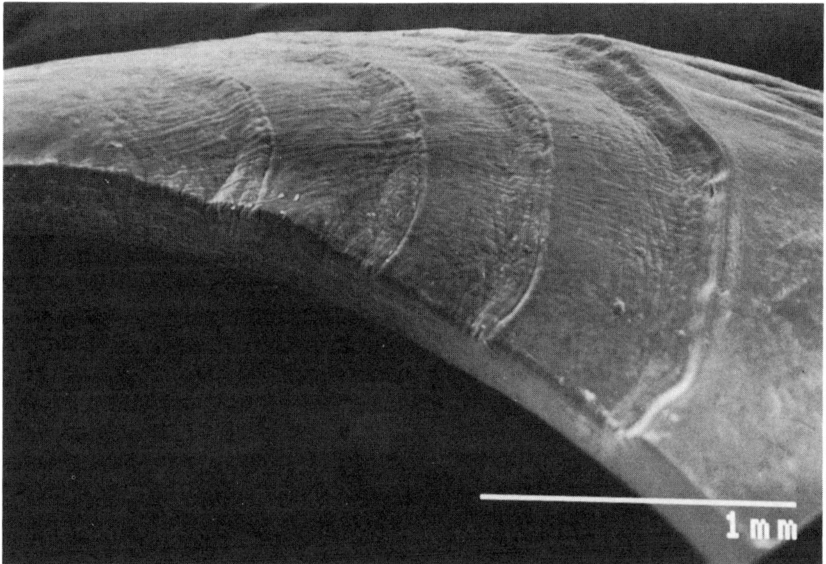


**Fig 9–5.**—Scanning electron micrograph of the ablated corneal surface. The margins of the ablations are not perfectly circular but formed of a series of straight lines. This has been caused by imaging the edges of the leaves of the aperture in the mechanical iris diaphragm through which the beam passed. (Courtesy of Marshall J, Trokel SL, Rothery S, et al: *Ophthalmology* 95:1411–1421, October 1988.)

seal the exposed surface. Endothelial damage does not occur. Further studies of the stability of induced refractive change are needed.

▶ Although precise ablation corneal surgery using an excimer laser is now feasible, we still do not know the results of long-term healing and subsequent visual acuity. This study in monkeys indicates that healing is slow and some minimal superficial stromal change exists even 8 months after the surgery. The visual acuity results are unknown, but studies such as these provide a background of knowledge for this new form of refractive surgery. Cautious optimism is the rule, with human application of this technique in experimental design the next step.—P.R. Laibson, M.D.

---

## Corneal Allograft Rejection Following Immunization

Steinemann TL, Koffler BH, Jennings CD (Univ of Kentucky; VA Hosps, Lexington, Ky)
*Am J Ophthalmol* 106:575–578, November 1988                    9–20

---

In 5 patients corneal allograft rejection occurred after immunization. One patient received a tetanus toxoid booster 9 months after corneal transplantation for keratoconus and rejection developed within 4 days. After 2 years, penetrating keratoplasty was necessary, but this graft became cloudy following hepatitis B immunization 6 months later. The other 4 patients experienced rejection after influenza immunization. Two were treated effectively with high-dose steroids. All of these rejection episodes occurred within several weeks of influenza immunization.

Immunization may lead to the expression and recognition of major histocompatibility complex antigens in the cornea. Viral syndromes are temporally associated with renal allograft rejection, and theoretically a similar stimulus for rejection could come from immunization via generalized T cell activation. Patients should know that immunization may pose a risk to their corneal transplants. Increased use of topical forms of steroids before and after immunization may protect the graft.

# 10 Retina

## Current Management of Postsurgical Endophthalmitis

WILLIAM E. BENSON, M.D.
*Cornea Department, Wills Eye Hospital, Philadelphia, Pennsylvania*

The past 12 years have seen a dramatic change in the management and visual prognosis of patients with endophthalmitis. Thirteen years ago the debate was over whether to use intravitreal antibiotics or to limit therapy to topical, periocular, and intravenous antibiotics (1,2). Today, intravitreal antibiotics are used routinely, and the advent of microsurgical techniques and intraocular instruments has had a significant influence on the management of the infected eye. The current debate revolves around the indications for vitrectomy and whether intravenous antibiotics are necessary at all. This introduction will discuss postsurgical endophthalmitis because it is the most common cause of endophthalmitis and is the diagnosis surgeons fear more than any other. A brilliant cataract operation may be spoiled by the unexpected infection of the eye.

### Diagnosis

I think that clinicians are getting better and better in diagnosing early endophthalmitis. Because they are aware that many infections develop after the cutting or removal of corneoscleral sutures (3), they follow these patients more closely. The most significant presenting symptoms are pain and precipitously decreased vision. The most important sign is hypopyon. Others include eyelid edema, chemosis, injection, corneal edema, marked cells and flare in the anterior chamber, and vitreous cells. In some cases it is difficult to differentiate severe postoperative uveitis from endophthalmitis because both may have all of the above mentioned signs and symptoms. A recently recognized ancillary test that is helpful in such cases is B-scan ultrasonography. If multiple echoes from numerous vitreous cells are present, the clinician should lean more toward the diagnosis of endophthalmitis. It is essential also to know that all of the above signs and symptoms are not present in every case. Patients with culture-proven infection have denied pain.

### The Role of Vitrectomy

Machemer's introduction of vitrectomy revolutionized the management of endophthalmitis. Theoretically, vitrectomy should help to cure endophthalmitis, because it is essentially the equivalent of draining an abscess. Vitrectomy removes large quantities of bacteria and bacterial debris, clears the ocular media, and permits better diffusion of antibiotics. In addition, it increases the likelihood of identifying the causative organism. Despite these considerations, it was an experimental study by Cottingham and Forster (4) that gave impetus to its widespread use. They injected a large inoculum of *Staphylococcus aureus* into the rabbit eye. Twenty-five hours later the animals were given intravitreal gentamicin alone, subjected to surgery (lensectomy and vitrectomy) alone, or were treated with both antibiotics and surgery. Gentamicin alone cured the infection in 33% of the eyes. Surgery alone cured 50% of the eyes if operative intervention was undertaken within 24 hours of the inoculum. Significantly, the combination of antibiotic and vitrectomy was effective in 83% of the eyes. The beneficial effect of vitrectomy was later confirmed by others (5,6).

Some experts (3,7,8) recommend that vitrectomy not be done in mild to moderate endophthalmitis, especially if the infection seems to begin 4 or more days postoperatively. The basis for this opinion is that the most common cause of postcataract surgery endophthalmitis is *Staphylococcus epidermidis,* and visual results without vitrectomy are as good or better as those with vitrectomy. Similarly, experimental *S. epidermidis* endophthalmitis can be cured by intravitreal antibiotics alone (4). The problem is how to be sure that a given infection is *S. epidermidis* and not a more virulent organism such as *S. aureus.* Endophthalmitis caused by these pathogens usually develops within 72 hours postoperatively. Unfortunately, this is not always true, however, and valuable time may be lost by deferring vitrectomy.

Unless the infection is mild, I and others (9) treat definite and probable endophthalmitis in the same way, especially if less than 1 week has passed since cataract surgery. It is essential to examine both the aqueous and the vitreous for infective organisms. Usually, the vitreous is much more likely to yield the causative organism than is the aqueous. On the other hand, the aqueous should not be neglected because, rarely, the vitreous specimen is negative and the aqueous positive. I almost never do a needle aspiration of the vitreous for three reasons: First, a "blind" vitreous tap may miss a focal vitreous abscess; second, it may cause severe traction on the vitreous base with retinal break formation; third, because vitrectomy probably causes no more complications than "blind" needle aspiration, it does not make sense to delay the definitive therapy.

Another advantage of prompt vitrectomy is that the eye is softened enough to permit antibiotic therapy immediately, which we begin as soon as the specimens for culture have been removed. The vitrectomy infusion fluid contains 8 mg of gentamicin per 1,000 ml (0.2 ml of gentamicin solution containing 40 mg/ml with 1 L of infusion fluid). At the end of surgery we inject gentamicin, 200 µg; cefazolin, 2.25 mg; and dexamethasone, 400 mg. Inadvertent injection of high doses of gentamicin has been reported by various authors to produce severe retinal ischemia and macular infarction. We prefer the surgeon to draw up antibiotics for intravitreal use before injection, or if prepared by the pharmacy, for the syringes to be clearly labeled and color coded.

## Should the Intraocular Lens Be Removed?

Initially, most surgeons removed the intraocular lens (IOL) as part of the surgery. Now, however, we do not recommend removal of the IOL. Such surgery not only is difficult and bloody, but it also removes any potential benefit the patient may receive once the inflammation has resolved. Experimental studies found that endophthalmitis can be cured without removing the IOL (10). In a recent clinical series, 56 of 57 eyes were sterilized with the lens in place (3). The exception is fungal endophthalmitis, when removal of the IOL and generous excision of the vitreous are mandatory.

## The Intravenous Use of Antibiotics Postoperatively

Until recently, most surgeons routinely treated patients with intravenous antibiotics postoperatively while awaiting culture results. Now even this has become controversial after the provocative paper by Pavan and Brinser (11) who treated 16 eyes with vitrectomy and several intravitreal injections of antibiotics but none systemically. All infections were eradicated with excellent visual results.

## *Propionibacterium* Endophthalmitis: Endophthalmitis Caused by Anerobic Bacteria

It has been recognized recently that anerobic bacteria, especially *Propionibacterium acnes* can cause endophthalmitis. Unlike that caused by aerobic bacteria, the infection usually develops weeks or months after cataract surgery (12,13). The diagnosis will not be made correctly unless careful anaerobic culture techniques are used. Patients may have a moderate or severe infection in the anterior chamber or hypopyon and thickening of the posterior capsule with "plaque" formation. They often do not have pain, severe injection, or chemosis. The correct management of these infections has yet to be determined. Initially, because the bacteria lurked under the capsule or in remaining cortical material, it was thought that removal of the IOL and complete removal of the posterior capsule with alpha-chymotrypsin was indicated. More recently, at Wills Eye Hospital we have begun to treat these patients with intravitreal and systemic antibiotics and without vitrectomy.

*References*

1. Baum JL: Antibiotic administration in the treatment of bacterial endophthalmitis. I. Periocular injections. *Surv Ophthalmol* 21:332–338, 1977.
2. Peyman GA: Antibiotic administration in the treatment of bacterial endophthalmitis. II. Intravitreal injections. *Surv Ophthalmol* 21:339–346, 1977.
3. Driebe WT, Mandelbaum S, Forster RK, et al: Pseudophakic endophthalmitis. Diagnosis and management. *Ophthalmology* 93:442–448, 1986.
4. Cottingham AJ, Forster RK: Vitrectomy in endophthalmitis. Results of

a study using vitrectomy, intraocular antibiotics, or a combination of both. *Arch Ophthalmol* 94:2078–2081, 1976.

5. McGetrick JJ, Peyman GA: Vitrectomy in experimental endophthalmitis: II. Bacterial endophthalmitis. *Ophthalmic Surg* 6:45–55, 1979.

6. Talley AR, D'Amico DJ, Talamo JH, et al: The role of vitrectomy in the treatment of postoperative bacterial endophthalmitis. *Arch Ophthalmol* 105:1699–1702, 1987.

7. O'Day DM, Jones DB, Patrinely J, et al: *Staphylococcus epidermidis* endophthalmitis: Visual outcome following noninvasive therapy. *Ophthalmology* 89:354–360, 1982.

8. O'Day DM: Medical treatment of endophthalmitis, in Spaeth GL, Katz LJ (eds): *Current Therapy in Ophthalmic Surgery*. Philadelphia, BC Decker, 1989, pp 344–347.

9. Ficker LA, Meredith TA, Wilson LA, et al: Role of vitrectomy in *Staphylococcus epidermidis*. *Br J Ophthalmol* 72:386–389, 1988.

10. Hopen G, Mondino BJ, Kozy D, et al: Intraocular lenses and experimental bacterial endophthalmitis. *Am J Ophthalmol* 94:402–407, 1982.

11. Pavan PR, Brinser JH: Exogenous bacterial endophthalmitis treated without systemic antibiotics. *Am J Ophthalmol* 104:121–126, 1987.

12. Meisler DM, Palestine AG, Vastine DW, et al: Chronic *Propionibacterium* endophthalmitis after extracapsular cataract extraction and intraocular lens implantation. *Am J Ophthalmol* 102:733–739, 1986.

13. Ormerod LD, Paton BG, Haaf J, et al: Anaerobic bacterial endophthalmitis. *Ophthalmology* 94:799–808, 1987.

**Early Vitrectomy for Severe Proliferative Diabetic Retinopathy in Eyes With Useful Vision: Results of a Randomized Trial—Diabetic Retinopathy Vitrectomy Study Report 3**

The Diabetic Retinopathy Vitrectomy Study Research Group (Natl Eye Inst, Bethesda, Md)

*Ophthalmology* 95:1307–1320, October 1988

10–1

A previous study assessed the risks and benefits of performing early pars plana vitrectomy in eyes with advanced proliferative diabetic retinopathy (PDR). A second clinical trial was undertaken to compare early vitrectomy with conventional management in eyes with extensive, active, neovascular or fibrovascular proliferations and useful vision. The series included 370 eyes with PDR, no central retinal detachment, and visual acuity of 10/200 or better. Patients were randomly assigned to receive either early vitrectomy or conventional management.

Eyes in the least severe new vessel severity (NVC) subgroup, of which half were barely eligible by photographic criteria and half were eligible only by clinical assessment, did not appear to benefit from early vitrectomy. In this subgroup eyes managed conventionally had a similar chance of good vision and a smaller risk of poor vision or no light perception than eyes undergoing early vitrectomy. Vitrectomy was needed in only 40% of conventionally managed eyes in this subgroup during the 4-year follow-up.

For eyes in the moderately severe NVC group, early vitrectomy seemed to increase the chance of good vision without increasing the risk of poor vision, but it was associated with a small rise in the proportion with no light perception. As in the least severe group, only 40% of conventionally treated eyes underwent vitrectomy.

In the severe and very severe groups, early vitrectomy provided a substantial increase in the chance of good vision and a corresponding decrease in the risk of poor vision at 3 and 4 years. There was little change in the risk of no light perception. The rate of vitrectomy in eyes treated conventionally was 35% in the severe group and 65% in the very severe group by the end of the first year of follow-up; at 4 years these rates were 50% and 85%, respectively.

Early vitrectomy should be considered in eyes with useful vision and advanced active PDR with extensive new vessels. The more severe the new vessels and the poorer the outlook for improvement with photocoagulation, the more seriously early vitrectomy should be considered.

► The proper timing for vitrectomy in PDR remains controversial. The most important information that this study presents is that patients with decreased vision caused by severe PDR have a 50% to 85% chance of requiring vitrectomy subsequently if they are treated with photocoagulation and observation alone. Eyes with only mild or moderate neovascularization have about a 40% chance of subsequently requiring vitrectomy. For patients with all levels of severity of neovascularization, those who had early vitrectomy had a 57% better chance of having final visual acuity of at least 20/40 than did those who were initially observed without vitrectomy. However, the same percentage of each group had acuity of 20/60 or better, indicating that the visual benefit of early vitrectomy in PDR is small. In summary, this study shows that the timing for vitrectomy must be individualized; there are no hard and fast rules as to which patient must have a vitrectomy.—W.E. Benson, M.D.

---

## A Clinical Comparison of Central and Peripheral Argon Laser Panretinal Photocoagulation for Proliferative Diabetic Retinopathy

Blankenship GW (Univ of Miami)
*Ophthalmology* 95:170–177, February 1988                    10–2

---

Fifty eyes having 3 or 4 risk factors for diabetic retinopathy received argon laser panretinal photocoagulation (PRP) in either a central or peripheral distribution. All of these eyes, with extensive neovascular proliferative retinopathy, were treated in the midperipheral fundus; half were treated more centrally and half were treated more peripherally.

One-fourth of the patients treated centrally lost at least 2 lines of acuity within 6 months after treatment compared with only 8% of those treated peripherally. The mean visual field constriction with the I–4e isopter was 39% after central treatment and 29% after peripheral PRP. For the IV–4e isopter the respective figures were 12% and 7%. Macular edema increased in 19% of centrally treated eyes but decreased in 19%

after peripheral PRP. Complete disk neovascular regression occurred in 38% of the centrally treated group and 47% of the peripherally treated group. Partial regression was obtained in 31% and 33% of eyes, respectively.

Both types of PRP yielded good results compared with other reports. However, it appears to be helpful to lower the amount of laser treatment in and about the posterior fundus during PRP. Loss of significant central acuity is less frequent with this type of treatment, as is macular edema, and neovascular proliferation regresses as well as with central treatment.

▶ This report suggests that for many patients, treatment close to the macula not only is not necessary but plays an important role in the increased macular edema seen after panretinal photocoagulation. In patients with macular edema, especially if they had loss of central vision after PRP in the fellow eye, this strategy should be considered.—W.E. Benson, M.D.

---

**Modified Grid Laser Photocoagulation for Diabetic Macular Edema: The Effect on the Central Visual Field**
Striph GG, Hart WM Jr, Olk RJ (Washington Univ)
*Ophthalmology* 95:1673–1679, December 1988

10–3

Visual acuity stabilizes in patients with diabetic macular edema after grid laser photocoagulation, but the effect on extrafoveal visual function is not clear. Automated static threshold perimetry was performed on 64 eyes of 36 patients before and after modified grid treatment with the argon green laser or the krypton red laser. Twenty-eight eyes were retreated because of persistent macular edema.

The average threshold sensitivity in the central 5 degrees declined by 3.4 dB after the first treatment and by 6.9 dB cumulatively after the second treatment. Gray-scale displays of the central field were darker after treatment, but scotomas resulting from treatment could not be distinguished from those resulting from macular edema. The foveal threshold did not change significantly after treatment. There was no apparent change in color vision. Comparable changes followed treatment with the 2 types of laser.

In modified grid laser photocoagulation visual acuity and foveal threshold are preserved in patients with diabetic macular edema at the cost of a generalized loss of threshold sensitivity across the central part of the visual field.

---

**Progression of Nonproliferative Diabetic Retinopathy Following Cataract Extraction**
Jaffe GJ, Burton TC (Med College of Wisconsin, Milwaukee)
*Arch Ophthalmol* 106:745–749, June 1988

10–4

Eight patients who had progressive nonproliferative diabetic retinopathy after cataract extraction were followed. Six underwent uncomplicated extracapsular extraction with placement of a posterior chamber intraocular lens. In the other 2, surgery was complicated by vitreous loss. Severe exudative macular edema developed in both patients, with diffuse retinal thickening, fluorescein leakage, increased dot and blot hemorrhages, and lipid deposition. All 8 patients had clinically meaningful macular edema in the operated-on eye. Six received laser photocoagulation. Final acuity was worse than preoperative acuity in 6 patients and was unchanged in the other 2. No patient had a final acuity better than 20/50. The fellow eyes were stable.

Aiello et al. reported that diabetics with proliferative retinopathy are at increased risk of neovascular glaucoma or rubeosis iridis developing after intracapsular cataract extraction. Patients with existing background retinopathy should know that cataract surgrey sometimes is followed by progression of retinopathy and loss of vision.

▶ The authors report a phenomenon well known to all retinal specialists and to many cataract surgeons. Usually, patients with diabetic macular edema who undergo cataract surgery have a worsening of the edema—even patients with uncomplicated extracapsular cataract extraction. Often, the edema regresses after a period of 6–12 months. Clearly, extreme caution is indicated in operating on these patients.—W.E. Benson, M.D.

---

## Progression of Diabetic Retinopathy After Pancreas Transplantation for Insulin-Dependent Diabetes Mellitus

Ramsay RC, Goetz FC, Sutherland DER, Maurer SM, Robison LL, Cantrill HL, Knoblock WH, Najarian JS (Univ of Minnesota)
*N Engl J Med* 318:208–214, Jan 28, 1988                                        10–5

---

Short-term benefits accrue to tighter metabolic control of insulin-dependent diabetes, but long-term clinical benefits remain to be documented. Intense insulin treatment carries its own problems. The ocular effects of successful pancreas transplantation and resultant normoglycemia were studied in 22 patients with type I diabetes using 16 patients in whom transplantation had failed as a control group. The respective mean hemoglobin $A_1$ levels were 7% and 12%. Most patients in both groups had advanced proliferative retinopathy at the outset.

Similar progression of retinopathy was evident in the 2 groups after a mean follow-up of 24 months. In both, progression was more frequent in patients with low baseline retinopathy scores. There may have been less deterioration in eyes with advanced changes after 3 years of euglycemia, but rates of visual loss were similar in both groups.

Maintenance of normoglycemia after successful pancreas transplantation does not prevent or reverse diabetic retinopathy in patients with insulin-dependent diabetes. Possibly, very early transplantation could prevent diabetic retinopathy if the diabetic state is totally reversed for a long period.

▶ Here is further proof that once diabetic retinopathy is established it may be too late to prevent progression by strict control of the blood glucose level. Whether control of the blood glucose level will prevent the development of retinopathy if instituted shortly after onset of diabetes remains to be proven. Most experimental and clinical studies indicate that it will.—W.E. Benson, M.D.

## Increased Ocular Blood Flow and $^{125}$I-Albumin Permeation in Galactose-Fed Rats: Inhibition by Sorbinil

Tilton RG, Chang K, Weigel C, Eades D, Sherman WR, Kilo C, Williamson JR (Washington Univ)
*Invest Ophthalmol Vis Sci* 29:861–868, June 1988          10–6

Many manifestations of diabetic eye disease, including cataracts, retinal capillary basement membrane thickening, and microaneurysms, appear to be aldose reductase-linked phenomena caused by the increased metabolism of glucose and galactose to their respective sugar alcohols, sorbitol and galactitol. Assessment was made of $^{125}$I-albumin permeation and blood flow, using $^{85}$Sr-labeled microspheres, in the eye and brain of rats fed a diet of 50% dextrin or 50% galactose.

Blood flow was increased in the retina, choroid, and anterior uvea of galactose-fed rats but not in the brain. It was normalized by sorbinil, an aldose reductase inhibitor. Permeation of labeled albumin was increased in the retina, choroid, and anterior uvea of galactose-fed rats but was unchanged in the brain. Sorbinil normalized albumin penetration in the ocular tissues in rats fed galactose for 8 months. Polyol levels also were increased in ocular tissues in rats given the galactose diet; sorbinil decreased but did not normalize these levels.

These findings support the concept that increased metabolism of hexoses to polyols, induced by diabetes or galactose ingestion, leads to impaired vascular hemodynamics and loss of barrier integrity. Smooth muscle cell contraction in resistance arterioles apparently is impaired by increased polyol metabolism. It was observed recently that diabetes-induced increases in ocular blood flow are prevented by aldose reductase inhibition.

▶ The ultimate prevention of diabetic retinopathy will come when a safe mechanism is discovered for maintaining blood sugar levels in the normal range. Until then, we must find ways to prevent the complications of hyperglycemia. The aldose reductase-sorbinil mechanism contributes to cataract formation in diabetics. This paper and others show a direct role in causation of retinopathy. Clinical trials of aldose reductase inhibitors are now underway.—W.E. Benson, M.D.

**Results and Complications of Pneumatic Retinopexy**
Chen JC, Robertson JE, Coonan P, Blodi CF, Klein ML, Watzke RC, Folk JC, Weingeist TA (Oregon Health Sciences Univ, Portland; Univ of Iowa)
*Ophthalmology* 95:601–608, May 1988                                           10–7

Pneumatic retinopexy is a means of avoiding a major surgical procedure for repairing retinal detachment, as well as the risks of general anesthesia. It often is done on an outpatient basis.

Fifty-one patients with primary rhegmatogenous retinal detachment underwent pneumatic retinopexy. Reattachment occurred within 1 operation in 63% of the patients. Seventy-four percent of 34 phakic eyes and 41% of 17 aphakic or pseudophakic eyes were reattached. New tears developed in 22% of treated eyes. Other complications included inadequate closure of the original tear, shifting and delayed absorption of subretinal fluid, and the opening of previously closed tears. One patient had a redetachment 9 months after the initial procedure, but the outcome was still considered a success. Proliferative vitreoretinopathy developed in 5 patients, 4 in the aphakic/pseudophakic group, and necessitated scleral buckle and vitrectomy to reattach the retina.

Pneumatic retinopexy is a promising alternative approach to primary rhegmatogenous retinal detachment, but there are many risks and complications. An increased rate of new tears was noted in the present series. Much less success is obtained in eyes with aphakic or pseudophakic detachment, and more careful patient selection is required in this group.

▶ The high failure rate of pneumatic retinopexy in aphakic and pseudophakic eyes is now well documented. The technique should be used only rarely in such patients. Even in phakic patients this technique remains highly controversial. At a recent meeting of the Retina Society, an overwhelming majority of retinal surgeons present stated that they would not have this technique used on them if they had a one-quadrant retinal detachment with the macula on.— W.E. Benson, M.D.

**Management of Anterior and Posterior Proliferative Vitreoretinopathy: XLV Edward Jackson Memorial Lecture**
Aaberg TM (Med College of Wisconsin, Milwaukee)
*Am J Ophthalmol* 106:519–532, November 1988                                   10–8

In proliferative vitreoretinopathy anterior and posterior proliferation produces multidirectional tractional forces. Pigment epithelial cells released after retinal detachment undergo metaplastic change and some become fibroblast-like cells that spread along adjacent ocular surfaces. Retinal astrocytes also have a role in the proliferative process.

Multiple radial incisions in the vitreous base serve to relax the circumferential traction created by anterior proliferation. Forward displacement of the vitreous base and associated anterior retina is eliminated by incising the displaced anterior and posterior hyaloid surfaces. Subsequently,

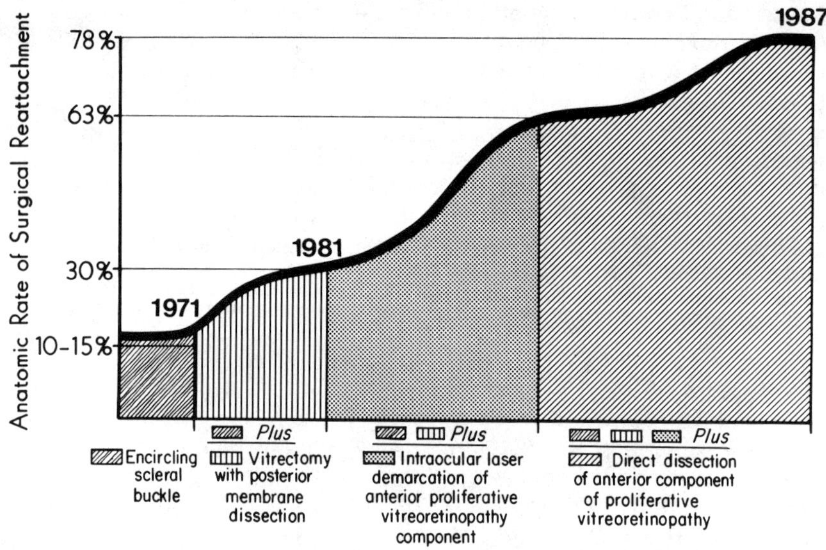


Fig 10–1.—Correlation of increasing rate of long-term retinal reattachment after surgery for proliferative vitreoretinopathy with innovations of surgical technology. (Courtesy of Aaberg TM: *Am J Ophthalmol* 106:519–532, November 1988.)

posterior traction is released and final tamponade is produced with gas or silicone oil.

Endolaser photocoagulation techniques have greatly expanded the application of vitreoretinal surgery. Internal drainage of subretinal fluid through a retinotomy now is possible. Retinal holes detected by the operating microscope can be treated.

Total retinal reattachment was achieved in 70% of 33 eyes with posterior proliferation only and in 57% of 47 eyes with significant anterior proliferation. Retinal attachment posterior to the scleral buckle was realized in 82% and 79% of eyes, respectively. These results reflect the significant advances made in recent years (Fig 10–1). There now are virtually no technically inoperable retinal detachments.

## Nuclear Sclerosis After Vitrectomy for Idiopathic Epiretinal Membranes

de Bustros S, Thompson JT, Michels RG, Enger C, Rice TA, Glaser BM (Johns Hopkins Univ; Yale Univ; Case Western Reserve Univ)
*Am J Ophthalmol* 105:160–164, February 1988                    10–9

Nuclear sclerotic lens changes can develop or progress after vitrectomy for epiretinal membranes affecting the macula, or "macular pucker." Seventy-five consecutive phakic eyes were examined after vitrectomy for macular pucker. Forty-seven percent of eyes had the appearance or progression of nuclear sclerosis postoperatively. Sclerosis was moderate in 14 eyes and severe in 4. There were no anterior subcapsular cataract changes, and only 3 eyes had posterior subcapsular changes.

The development or progression of nuclear sclerosis after surgery was related to the presence of nuclear sclerosis preoperatively, the length of follow-up, and the surgeon. However, the differences between surgeons largely reflected differences in preoperative nuclear sclerosis and in length of follow-up. Life-table analysis of 53 eyes and fellow eyes showed significantly more nuclear sclerosis after surgery.

Nuclear sclerosis is a progressive change that worsens over time. Why it is a prominent postoperative observation is unclear, but this has important implications, particularly when vitrectomy is used as an option and in the treatment of primary rhegmatogenous retinal detachment.

▶ The high incidence of cataract after vitrectomy is yet another reason why this operation should never be undertaken lightly. The authors' results suggest that vitrectomy should be used in primary scleral buckling procedures only in very selected cases.—W.E. Benson, M.D.

---

**Cystoid Macular Edema Following Extracapsular Cataract Extraction and Posterior Chamber Intraocular Lens Implantation**
Bradford JD, Wilkinson CP, Bradford RH Jr (Univ of Oklahoma)
*Retina* 8:161–164, 1988                                                      10–10

---

The course of clinical cystoid macular edema (CME) is good after cataract extraction in aphakic eyes without vitreous adhesions to the surgical wound, but the outcome is not as good in pseudophakic eyes with iris-fixated and iridocapsular intraocular lenses. Modern techniques of extracapsular cataract extraction with posterior chamber lens implantation are associated with a relatively low incidence of postoperative angiographic CME. The course of clinical CME after posterior chamber lens implantation was investigated.

In 20 symptomatic eyes extracapsular cataract extraction and posterior chamber intraocular lens implantation were done. Resolution of the symptomatic clinical CME was noted in 90% of the eyes. In those that ultimately resolved, clearing was observed within the first 12 months in 78% and within 24 months in 94%. Of the 7 eyes with a primary posterior capsulotomy, 86% experienced resolution of CME, as did 92% of the 13 eyes with an intact capsule. Visual acuity returned to 20/40 or better in the eyes in which CME resolved.

These findings suggest that clinical CME in patients with a posterior chamber intraocular lens has a relatively favorable course. Ninety percent of the 20 eyes in this series had resolution of CME.

▶ This article strongly suggests that the course of CME in patients with a posterior chamber lens is considerably better than that after intracapsular cataract extraction, with or without anterior chamber lenses. If the results can be corroborated by larger studies, the implication is that we should not rush into vitrectomy or other dramatic therapies but should wait for spontaneous resolution. Of course, acetazolamide (Diamox) may hasten the resolution of CME in selected cases. (See also Abstract 10–11.)—W.E. Benson, M.D.

## Treatment of Chronic Macular Edema With Acetazolamide
Cox SN, Hay E, Bird AC (Moorfields Eye Hosp, London)
*Arch Ophthalmol* 106:1190–1195, September 1988

10–11

The constant outward movement of fluid from the retina toward the choroid results in part from active transport of ions by the retinal pigment epithelium from its apical to basal surface with a consequent movement of water. This may be responsible for the relative deturgescence and ionic constancy of the outer retinal extracellular space. Pigment epithelial carbonic anhydrase enzyme systems are probably important in regulating ion transport. In induced nonrhegmatogenous retinal detachment in rabbit eyes, acetazolamide increases the rate of subretinal fluid reabsorption. In a prospective trial, 41 patients with chronic macular edema from various causes were given acetazolamide sodium, a carbonic anhydrase inhibitor.

Each patient received a 5-cycle crossover regimen of treatment or no treatment, with another 2 cycles of crossover with cyclopenthiazide, a diuretic that does not inhibit carbonic anhydrase. The best predictor of response was the cause of the disease. In the 2 groups with retinal venous obstruction, none of the patients responded to treatment; but more than half of those with inflammatory and genetically determined disorders had a good response.

These data have therapeutic implications. The macular edema associated with retinitis pigmentosa may add greatly to overall visual disability. Aphakic macular edema is common but usually self-limiting. Acetazolamide may prove helpful in the small number of cases that do not resolve.

▶ This is truly an exciting article. The authors took a drug with which we have considerable clinical experience and used it to treat several refractory conditions. I have already begun to try this in selected patients, and although some did not respond, others have had dramatic improvement in vision. As the authors point out, acetazolamide may prove to be the best initial choice for the treatment of aphakic cystoid macular edema, intermediate uveitis, and retinitis pigmentosa.—W.E. Benson, M.D.

## A Clinical Index for Predicting Visual Acuity After Cataract Surgery
Graney MJ, Applegate WB, Miller ST, Elam JT, Freeman JM, Wood TO, Gettlefinger TC (Univ of Tennessee)
*Am J Ophthalmol* 105:460–465, May 1988

10–12

Patients with coincident retinal disease who are undergoing cataract surgery are at increased risk for an unsuccessful outcome. Thus clinicians must be able to identify patients with retinal disease that might limit postoperative visual acuity. A clinical index for predicting postoperative visual acuity in cataract patients was developed and cross-validated using data from 182 patients aged 70 years and older.

Four predictor variables were considered practical for widespread clinical use and correlated statistically with postoperative visual acuity: age, preoperative Snellen visual acuity, number of current prescription medications used, and newspaper reading. This index was 72% accurate in predicting postoperative visual acuity within 1 Snellen line for patients undergoing cataract surgery. Further analysis showed the clinical index to be more accurate than 2 sophisticated instruments used to predict postoperative visual acuity: a laser interferometer and a potential acuity meter.

Media opacity that militates against ophthalmoscopic evaluation of the fundus also seems to impair technical instrument assessment. Technical instrument retinal visual acuity measurements of 0.50 or more predicted success correctly 90% of the time; however, the instruments' retinal visual acuity measurements below 0.50 were not predictive of surgical outcome in 3 of every 4 patients predicted to be at increased risk for surgical failure. Negative predictions were more reliably obtained with the clinical index. Two of every 3 predictions below 0.50 obtained using the clinical index were correct predictions of failure.

This clinical index developed to predict postoperative visual acuity in cataract patients was 72% accurate in predicting surgical outcome within 1 Snellen line. The index was more accurate than 2 sophisticated instruments used to predict postoperative visual acuity.

▶ In this age of high-tech ophthalmology, it is comforting to know that 4 simply measured predictor variables can outperform expensive instrumentation. The main problem with the expensive instrumentation is that it frequently is not helpful in exactly the patients for whom we need the information. I place more faith in a careful slit-lamp and fundus examination than I do in the laser interferometer and the potential acuity meter.—W.E. Benson, M.D.

---

## Long-Term Follow-Up of a Prospective Trial of Argon Laser Photocoagulation in the Treatment of Central Serous Retinopathy

Ficker L, Vafidis G, While A, Leaver P (Moorfields Eye Hosp, London)
*Br J Ophthalmol* 72:829–834, November 1988                    10–13

---

Argon laser photocoagulation was evaluated in a series of 69 patients with central serous retinopathy in 70 eyes. During follow-up from 6½ to 12 years there was no evidence that treatment significantly influenced the visual outcome, as measured by the Snellen chart and the Farnsworth-Munsell 100-hue discrimination test.

Treatment did not reduce the recurrence note or the prevalence of chronic disease (Fig 10–2). More than 40% of treated patients had an-

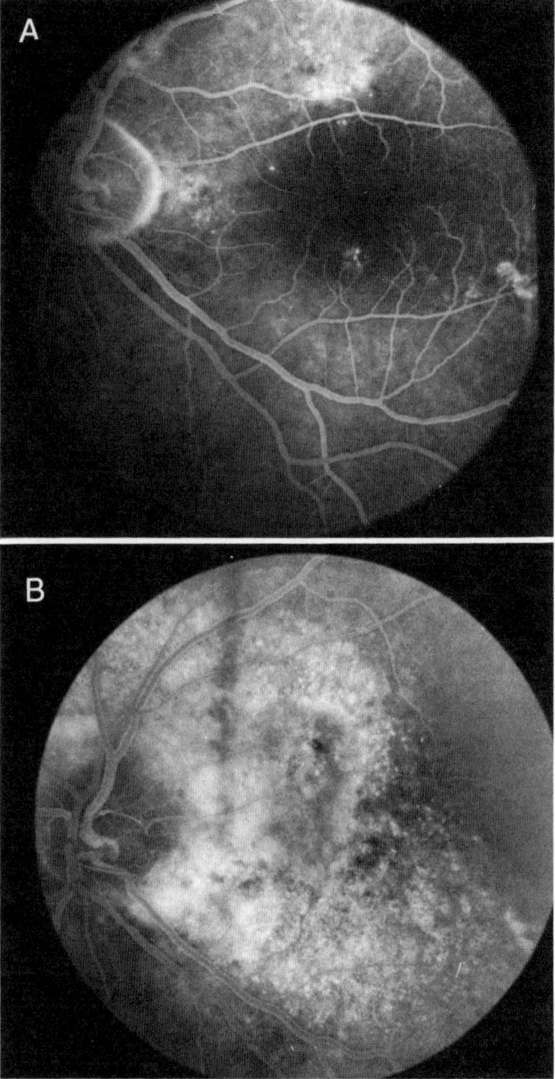

Fig 10–2.—**A,** resolution of central serous retinopathy after treated recurrence. **B,** progressive retinal pigment epithelial disturbance 8 years after treatment. (Courtesy of Ficker L, Vafidis G, While A, et al: *Br J Ophthalmol* 72:829–834, November 1988.)

giographically documented recurrences. Nevertheless, the long-term visual outcome was good.

Argon laser photocoagulation appears not to lower the risk of chronic central serous retinopathy. Progressive retinal pigment epithelial disease does pose a threat of permanent visual loss, but photocoagulation is indicated only to relieve symptoms in patients with good acuity. Treatment can hasten resolution of serous detachment.

## Natural Course of Poorly Defined Choroidal Neovascularization Associated With Macular Degeneration

Bressler NM, Frost LA, Bressler SB, Murphy RP, Fine SL (Johns Hopkins Univ)
*Arch Ophthalmol* 106:1537–1542, November 1988                  10–14

The natural course of age-related macular degeneration was studied in 84 eyes with poorly defined angiographic leakage, which was presumed to reflect choroidal neovascularization. The patients, all older than age 50 years, had subsensory retinal fluid in the macula and multiple areas of hyperfluorescence that were more intense in later phases of the angiogram, with leakage in the middle and late phases.

Average initial visual acuity was 20/80. Leakage involved the foveal center of the outset in 89% of eyes. After an average follow-up of 28 months the average acuity was 20/250. In 42% of eyes the acuity declined by at least 6 lines. In only 14% of eyes did the final acuity remain the same or improve. Sixty-one percent of eyes had diskiform scars at last assessment. Thirty-three percent continued to have poorly defined leakage without evidence of scarring. One eye had geographic atrophy without leakage or scarring.

It seems possible that poorly defined neovascular membranes are a major cause of severe visual loss in elderly persons. Some eyes, however, do retain visual acuity or even improve. Severe visual loss correlates with the development of diskiform scarring.

---

## Oral Zinc in Macular Degeneration

Newsome DA, Swartz M, Leone NC, Elston RC, Miller E (Louisiana State Univ; Univ of Utah, Logan; Utah State Univ, Logan)
*Arch Ophthalmol* 106:192–198, February 1988                  10–15

Macular degeneration associated with aging and drusen is the prime cause of severe visual loss in the United States and western Europe in those aged 55 and older. Laser photocoagulation does not benefit most persons with nonexudative disease. A double-blind, placebo-controlled

Change in Vision by Randomization Group*

| Outcome | Zinc-Treated Group (n = 80) | Placebo Group (n = 71) | Total (N = 151) |
|---|---|---|---|
| | **Frequency (%)** | | |
| Gain of ≥ 10 letters | 3 (3.75) | 1 (1.41) | 4 (2.65) |
| Change of ± 9 or fewer letters | 66 (82.50) | 46 (64.79) | 112 (74.17) |
| Loss of 10 to 14 letters | 5 (6.25) | 13 (18.31) | 18 (11.92) |
| Loss of 15 to 19 letters | 4 (5.00) | 6 (8.45) | 10 (6.62) |
| Loss of ≥ 20 letters | 2 (2.50) | 5 (7.04) | 7 (4.64) |
| **Total** | **80 (100)** | **71 (100)** | **151 (100)** |

*Data obtained from 1 eye in patients were pooled with those obtained from 2 eyes.
(Courtesy of Newsome DA, Swartz M, Leone NC, et al: *Arch Ophthalmol* 106:192–198, February 1988.)

study was made of oral zinc therapy in 151 patients with drusen or macular degeneration. High concentrations of zinc normally are present in the retina and pigment epithelium, which are involved in the disease process. Treated patients received 100 mg of zinc sulfate in tablet form.

Some eyes in the zinc-treated group lost vision, but the group as a whole had significantly less visual loss than the patients given placebo after 1–2 years (table). This is the first controlled oral intervention study showing a positive, albeit limited, treatment effect in macular degeneration. Widespread use of zinc awaits further studies of toxic effects and complications. Dietary zinc is deficient to some degree in the diets of at least some groups at risk for the development of macular degeneration. The public health importance of this prevalent disorder justifies further trials of zinc therapy.

▶ It will be wonderful if the results of this study can be confirmed. If zinc or any other agent can be proven conclusively to prevent age-related macular degeneration, blindness in many patients might be prevented. Patients with a strong family history of macular degeneration might go on treatment early in life.—W.E. Benson, M.D.

---

**Visual Symptoms Associated With the Presence of a Lupus Anticoagulant**
Levine SR, Crofts JW, Lesser GR, Floberg J, Welch KMA (Henry Ford Hosp, Detroit; Univ of Michigan)
*Ophthalmology* 95:686–692, May 1988                    10–16

Lupus anticoagulant is an acquired serum immunoglobulin that prolongs several coagulation parameters, especially the partial thromboplastin time. Most often it is found in systemic lupus, but it also may occur with other collagen–vascular diseases and in otherwise healthy persons. The lupus anticoagulant has been associated with thrombosis despite laboratory findings suggesting impaired coagulation.

Five patients with lupus anticoagulant had branch retinal artery occlusion, ischemic optic neuropathy, transient visual loss, transient diplopia, and vertebrobasilar insufficiency, respectively. No treatment has consistently prevented recurrent thrombosis or symptoms in patients with the lupus anticoagulant. Treatment with steroids and anticoagulants, rather than antiplatelet agents alone, is recommended to prevent recurrent thrombosis in these patients. Treatment probably should continue for at least 3–6 months or until the partial thromboplastin time is normal. Refractory patients may receive immunosuppressive therapy.

Lupus anticoagulant should be considered in patients having retinal artery occlusion, ischemic optic neuropathy, or transient visual loss or diplopia. Recognition is especially important in young and middle-aged persons not otherwise at high risk of stroke. Lupus anticoagulant may be screened for using the VDRL, partial thromboplastin time, platelet count, and related anticardiolipin antibodies.

▶ Recent papers on the lupus anticoagulant factor represent further progress in our understanding of vascular obstructions in young persons. Although emboli and atherosclerosis account for most obstructions, clinicians must keep in mind other possibilities such as cardiac abnormalities, migraine, and the lupus anticoagulant.—W.E. Benson, M.D.

**Cryopexy of the Vitreous Base in the Management of Peripheral Uveitis**
Devenyi RG, Mieler WF, Lambrou FH, Will BR, Aaberg TM (Med College of Wisconsin, Milwaukee; Emory Univ)
*Am J Ophthalmol* 106:135–138, August 1988                    10–17

Since peripheral uveitis was first described more than 40 years ago, there have been limited advances in its treatment. A retrospective study examined eyes with peripheral uveitis resistant to conventional corticosteroid therapy that had vitreous base neovascularization and were treated with cryopexy. There were 27 affected eyes in 18 patients.

When cryopexy was applied to areas of active neovascularization, retrobulbar injection of lidocaine or general anesthesia was given, depending on the patient's age. Cryopexy, administered over the involved region of the vitreous base using indirect ophthalmoscopy, consisted of freezing, thawing, and refreezing. Usually, a conjunctival incision was not needed. All regions of neovascularization were treated, as well as adjacent areas containing dense exudate that were presumed to have underlying neovascularization. Uninvolved ciliary body and retina were treated 1 probe width beyond neovascularization.

Eighty-five percent of the eyes needed only 1 treatment, 11% needed 2, and 4% needed 3 treatments before regression of active neovascularization was achieved. At the last follow-up visit, 78% of the eyes were quiet, 18% had mild persistent inflammation, and 4% eventually atrophied.

The exact mechanism of action of cryopexy is not known. It does not treat the underlying cause of pars planitis; the rationale for such ablative treatment is to eliminate the neovascular and ischemic tissue. Eliminating this tissue may result in a decrease in exudate accumulation. In eyes with inflammation and vitreous base neovascularization, 78% treated with cryopexy became quiescent and remained stable without evidence of further disease progression.

▶ This study elaborates on previous work done at the Medical College of Wisconsin and strongly indicates that cryotherapy is beneficial in patients with peripheral uveitis. If corticosteroids cannot control the inflammation, cryotherapy is an excellent alternative.—W.E. Benson, M.D.

**Monitoring Communications Between Photoreceptors and Pigment Epithelial Cells: Effects of "Mild" Systemic Hypoxia**
Steinberg RH (Univ of California, San Francisco)
*Invest Ophthalmol Vis Sci* 28:1888–1904, December 1987          10–18

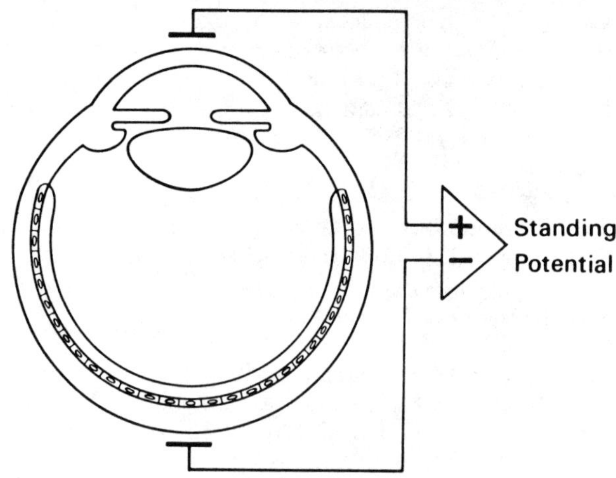


**Fig 10–3.**—Recording the standing potential of the eye. The standing potential can be recorded with DC amplification between an electrode on the cornea and a distant reference electrode. In darkness the standing potential is a steady-potential difference that has a positive polarity at the cornea. (Courtesy of Steinberg RH: *Invest Ophthalmol Vis Sci* 28:1888–1904, December 1987.)

Electrophysiologic methods are available to monitor communications between photoreceptors and retinal pigment epithelium (RPE) cells. Because the electrical activity of the RPE is practically intact at the cornea, recordings at the cornea provide a noninvasive means of studying RPE-photoreceptor interactions in the normal and diseased eye (Fig 10–3). Changes in blood oxygen alone alter the standing potential. For prac-

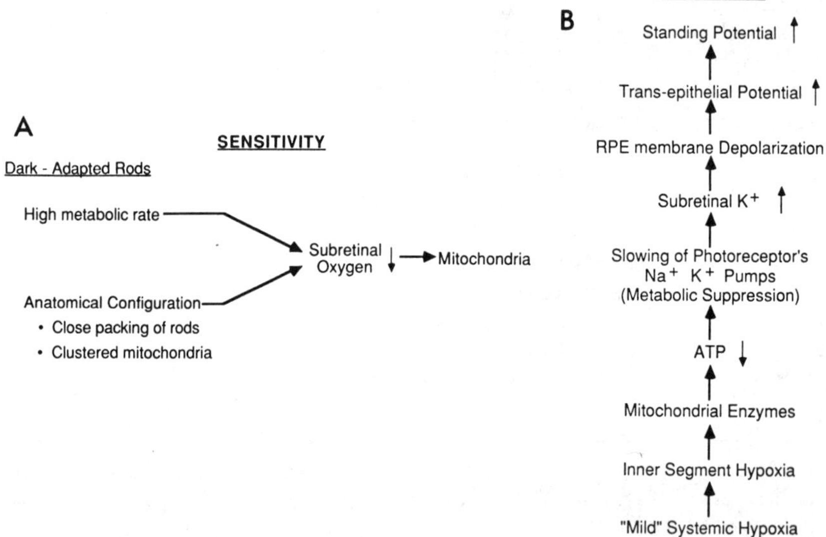


**Fig 10–4.**—Diagrammatic summaries of (**A**) hypothesis for sensitivity of rods in cat to "mild" systemic hypoxia, and (**B**) mechanism producing the increase in standing potential. (Courtesy of Steinberg RH: *Invest Ophthalmol Vis Sci* 28:1888–1904, December 1987.)

tical purposes, the potential is generated almost entirely by the epithelium, not by the neural retina. Depolarization of the RPE caused by mild hypoxia is accompanied by a substantial increase in subretinal $K^+$.

During maintained illumination, reaccumulation of potassium results chiefly from slowing of the $Na^+$-$K^+$ pump, and the reaccumulation permits study of the activity of the pump. Hypoxia in the dark retards or prevents the reaccumulation of $K^+$ during light, and light counters the hypoxic accumulation of $K^+$. Elevation of the $K^+$ concentration in the subretinal space causes the depolarization.

The high metabolic rate of rods in the dark, along with their anatomical configuration, brings the regional oxygen level to borderline hypoxia for mitochrondrial respiration (Fig 10–4). In mild systemic hypoxia, a further decrease in subretinal oxygen tension should lower the ATP supply of the rods and slow the $Na^+K^+$ pump. Sensing of hypoxia in the dark may be a protective mechanism that allows the rods to resist the damaging effects of hypoxia during complete dark adaptation when they are most vulnerable. The sensing process is an example of metabolic suppression. In a sense, light protects the rods from the effects of hypoxia. If disease overcomes the protective mechanism, the rods in the dark will be particularly sensitive to any interruption of their oxygen supply.

▶ Pursuit of the unexpected finding of a hypoxia-induced increase in the standing potential of the eye led to better understanding of the complex metabolic interactions in the retina. Such research may contribute to better understanding of retinal dystrophies.—W.E. Benson, M.D.

---

**Intravitreal Ganciclovir in the Treatment of AIDS-Associated Cytomegalovirus Retinitis**
Ussery FM III, Gibson SR, Conklin RH, Piot DF, Stool EW, Conklin AJ (Park Plaza Hosp, Houston)
*Ophthalmology* 95:640–648, May 1988                    10–19

---

Cytomegalovirus (CMV) retinitis is the most frequent opportunistic ocular infection in patients with acquired immunodeficiency syndrome (AIDS), reported in as many as 45% of patients during the average 20-month course. The only drug available that is effective against CMV retinitis is the antiviral agent ganciclovir.

Ganciclovir was injected into the vitreous in 14 eyes of 11 patients with severe AIDS-associated CMV retinitis. Six patients had progressive disease despite maximum intravenous doses of ganciclovir, whereas 5 had serious myelosuppression from intravenous treatment. Retinitis was suppressed in 78% of the treated eyes. The only complication was rhegmatogenous retinal detachment during 1 injection. Repeat injections were necessary in 9 eyes. Ophthalmoscopy was the best means of monitoring the response to intravitreal injections. Snellen acuities did not always reflect significant changes in the retinal status, and perimetry also was of limited use. Six of 7 eyes treated only intravitreally improved or stabilized.

In 10 of 11 eyes that were followed adequately acuity was maintained or improved after intravitreal ganciclovir therapy. It remains difficult to distinguish between the effects of the intravitreal and intravenous administration of ganciclovir in these cases. Nevertheless, intravitreal treatment appears to be effective and relatively safe, and provides an approach to myelosuppressed patients and those with breakthrough retinitis.

▶ With the increasing incidence of AIDS, blindness from CMV retinitis is becoming a common problem in many cities. Intravenous ganciclovir, the currently accepted therapy, is not satisfactory because of the severe neutropenia and thrombocytopenia it causes. Although repetaed intravitreal injections may also cause morbidity, this innovative treatment may preserve vision in many patients.—W.E. Benson, M.D.

---

**Ocular Toxoplasmosis in Patients With the Acquired Immunodeficiency Syndrome**
Holland GN, Engstrom RE Jr, Glasgow BJ, Berger BB, Daniels SA, Sidikaro Y, Harmon JA, Fischer DH, Boyer DS, Rao NA, Eagle RC Jr, Kreiger AE, Foos RY (Univ of California, Los Angeles; Univ of Texas, San Antonio; Wills Eye Hosp, Philadelphia; Univ of Southern California)
*Am J Ophthalmol* 106:653–667, December 1988                    10–20

---

Data were reviewed on presumed toxoplasmic retinochoroiditis in 8 patients with acquired immunodeficiency syndrome (AIDS) seen at 4 centers. In 7 the diagnosis was supported by a reduction or elimination of intraocular inflammation and healing of necrotic retinal lesions with antiparasitic drug therapy, in which pyrimethamine, sulfadiazine, clindamycin, tetracycline, and spiramycin were used. In 2 patients the diagnosis was confirmed histologically.

There was no evidence in these patients that the disease arose in preexisting retinochoroidal scars. Bilateral, multifocal lesions often were present. Vitreous inflammation was common, but there was little retinal inflammation in areas of necrosis. Two of 3 patients had reactivated, progressive disease after treatment was stopped. Retinal necrosis produced retinal tears or detachment in 3 patients. In 4 of 5 patients with multisystem involvement the ocular lesions were the initial manifestation of *Toxoplasma gondii* infection.

Ocular toxoplasmosis probably resulted from newly acquired infection or from dissemination of organisms from nonocular sites of disease. Inflammation tends to be prominent except in the retina, but hemorrhage is minimal. An accurate early diagnosis may allow medical treatment to preserve vision.

---

**Results and Prognostic Factors in Penetrating Ocular Injuries With Retained Intraocular Foreign Bodies**

Williams DF, Mieler WF, Abrams GW, Lewis H (Med College of Wisconsin, Milwaukee)
*Ophthalmology* 95:911–916, July 1988                                    10–21

Data were reviewed concerning 105 eyes with ocular injuries that involved retained intraocular foreign bodies. The patients were seen between 1977 and 1986, and were followed for at least 6 months (21 months on average). Sixty percent of the eyes had a final acuity of 20/40 or better, but 14% had vision worse than 5/200 and 6% of the eyes were enucleated.

A final acuity of 20/40 or better was most likely when initial acuity was at this level and when only 1 or 2 operations were needed. A wound 4 mm or more in length predicted poor final acuity. Most eyes were injured by hammering metal on metal. Five patients were wearing safety glasses at the time of injury. Sixty-five eyes had 1 operation only, and 28 other eyes had 2 procedures. Vitrectomy was the most frequent initial procedure. The route of foreign body removal did not determine visual outcome. Vitrectomy was most likely to be done in eyes with cataract, vitreous hemorrhage, or retinal tears.

Vitreous microsurgery has revolutionized the management of severe ocular injuries, including those with retained posterior segment foreign bodies. The rate of enucleation has declined because of the use of both vitrectomy and intraocular antibiotics. Vitrectomy may save some eyes that previously would have been removed. It also may help in the treatment of secondary complications such as proliferative vitreoretinopathy.

▶ In this study of 105 ocular injuries with retained intraocular foreign bodies, only 5 patients were wearing safety glasses at the time of injury. Certainly, more can be done to educate our patients about using protective glasses during times when they are at risk for severe eye injuries. Needless to say, multiple operations were required in many patients, and the visual outcome was directly related to the number of operations and size of the initial injury. No matter how bad the injury may seem, an attempt should be made to repair a severe anterior segment laceration with vitreous and/or iris and lens in the wound. I have been surprised at the good visual results sometimes achieved in what appear to be lost eyes.—P.R. Laibson, M.D.

**Temporary Keratoprosthesis for Combined Penetrating Keratoplasty, Pars Plana Vitrectomy, and Repair of Retinal Detachment**
Gelender H, Vaiser A, Snyder WB, Fuller DG, Hutton WL (Cornea Associates of Texas, Dallas; Texas Retina Associates, Dallas)
*Ophthalmology* 95:897–901, July 1988                                    10–22

Corneal opacity makes posterior segment surgery impossible in retinal detachment or vitreous hemorrhage. The Landers-Foulks temporary keratoprosthesis permits retinal and vitreous surgery in the presence of significant corneal opacity. At surgery the prosthesis is replaced by a homograft penetrating keratoplasty.

In 13 eyes with an opaque cornea and posterior segment abnormalities, a temporary keratoprosthesis was used to combine penetrating keratoplasty, pars plana vitrectomy, and scleral buckling. Trauma precipitated ocular disease in 7 eyes, whereas 6 patients had complications of cataract surgery. Some patients had endolaser photocoagulation or intraocular gas instillation. Three patients required lensectomy. In all cases the surgical plan was achieved successfully, and no untoward intraoperative complications occurred. In 8 eyes the retinal detachment was successfully reattached, but in 5 eyes the retina redetached as the eyes became phthisical. Visual function improved in 6 eyes. Injured eyes generally had a much poorer outcome than did eyes with problems related to cataract surgery.

The temporary keratoprosthesis allows attempted ocular repair in eyes that might otherwise not be approachable surgically. Vitreous complications can be treated effectively in conjunction with corneal transplant surgery without adversely affecting the state of the retina.

▶ Visual results with the temporary keratoprosthesis for severely traumatized eyes is very discouraging; although 1 patient did have 20/20 vision, the follow-up was only 9 months and one wonders what the ultimate vision will be. Surgeons performing this major combined anterior and posterior approach should be well versed in the numerous complications that can occur.—P.R. Laibson, M.D.

# 11 Visual Physiology

---

## Physiology, Refraction, Nystagmus, and Socioeconomic Issues

Robert D. Reinecke, M.D.
*Foerderer Eye Movement Center for Children, Wills Eye Hospital, Philadelphia, Pennsylvania*

In my first year as a reviewer for the Year Book of Ophthalmology a number of salient articles were identified that are important scientifically and are included for your perusal in the following pages. No socioeconomic issues were included, hence, the main item of this introduction will be on the Hsiao study. The major event for all of ophthalmology (and, indeed, perhaps all of medicine) has been the publication of the Hsiao report on the Resource-Based Relative Value Scale (RBRVS). This proposal to restructure physician fees has far-reaching implications for the manner in which ophthalmology is structured. I will review the theoretical basis for the Hsiao study, consider its implications on the structure of ophthalmological care, and discuss some shortcomings of the Hsiao study and the governmental structure where the debate on this issue will likely arise.

### Theoretical Basis for the Hsiao RBRVS

Few would argue that the physician reimbursement methodology for physician services under Medicare has many deficiencies. Experienced physicians have found themselves receiving lower fees than the new physician fresh from residency training. Discrepancies between fees given for the same procedure in differing geographical areas have been documented to be as great as 1 log unit. Some fees have emerged that are so low that physicians often do not even bill Medicare, as the overhead of billing is greater than the governmental fee. Some fees are substantial, particularly surgical fees. This disparity between the surgical fees and the internist's fees have caused the nonsurgical physicians to look for an alternative to the current "usual and customary." They believe that their manna has arrived in the RBRVS, which sets out as its goal to remedy disparities in fees between the surgeons and nonsurgeons. It is thus no surprise that the surgeons find the Hsiao study faulty and the nonsurgeons love it.

Both groups and Dr. Hsiao miss the point, however, that the government has little regard as to how the Medicare dollars are split between the physician groups, which is what the RBRVS is all about. Rather, it is looking for ways to cut its expenses of delivering medical care to the elderly. Interestingly, the RBRVS can be used to do that, namely, anything that any study, including the Hsiao study, offers that suggests any physician is being overcompensated for a procedure will surely be used to ratchet down that allowed reimbursement.

Unfortunately for the internists and rural practitioners, the Hsiao study will not be a vehicle for increased rates; rather, it will be used to cut the rates of reimbursement. Our government is currently spending 12.5% of its gross national product on medical care, and few supporters are urging more dollars to go into the medical care system. Thus the physicians are not only competing among themselves for the Medicare dollar, but also are competing with hospitals, nursing homes, and all other health care workers for their share of the pie.

The RBRVS will be an important document in the medical field and may end up having a tremendous impact on the delivery of medical care in the United States. In fact, it is likely to be the principal reason that we will have a flat fee structure in the next few years and probably will not be allowed any supplemental charges for the Medicare patient, even if that patient is a multimillionaire. The 1990s will be exciting!

The fundamental premise of the RBRVS structure is that physicians should be reimbursed equally for time delivering medical care if (1) the stress (intensity) to the physician, (2) the overhead, and (3) the training are all equal for a given service. It specifically excludes factors concerning (1) benefit to the patient, (2) the varying expertise of the physician, (3) quality of the service, (4) severity of the illness, and (5) supply and demand for the services. Thus the formula for the RBRVS is the estimation of total work multiplied by a factor for relative speciality costs. The latter include differences among specialities with respect to overhead expenses and professional liability costs (and the reports seem to indicate that a fudge factor is included that is specific for each specialty—more about that later). That product is further multiplied by the "amortized cost of specialty training," which is to account for the varying lengths of residencies.

The total work includes intraservice work and pre- and postservice work. The intraservice work consists of actual contact with the patient or the procedural time. Pre- and postservice work includes reviewing records and dictating charts. It should include the postoperative visits that are included in the global fee, but Hsiao has not done that for cataract surgery—a glaring omission in my view. Thus the RBRV may be written as follows:

$$RBRV = (TW) \times (1 + RPC) \times (1 + AST)$$

TW, total work by the physician.

RPC, index of relative specialty practice costs and ? malpractice costs.

AST, index of amortized value for the opportunity costs of specialized training.

The AST, or amortized specialty training costs, is factored out over the estimated professional life of the physician, thus variances in the time of training of 4 vs. 5 years post medical school are minor. The RPC, or relative practice costs, is calculated by Hsiao based on 1983 data. The change in office equipment for the ophthalmologist since that time is probably significant and should be updated. If corrections are applied here it would increase the index for ophthalmologists to a modest extent. Most of the difference in the RBRV is involved in the TW, or total work.

The work for a procedure was calculated in a somewhat round-about manner. First, four ophthalmologists agreed on 23 procedures that spanned the range of complexity and intensity of ophthalmologic services; a single service was given a score of 100, against which to judge all other services in comparison. For ophthalmology the service chosen to represent 100 was a chalazion incision and curettage. The value of 100 was unfortunate with respect to the chalazion as 100 is approximately the cost in dollars that many ophthalmologists charge for this procedure, thus all the other procedures were subconsciously indexed against their dollar charge background. These 23 procedures were enumerated in a survey sent to about 100 ophthalmologists; they were interviewed about the time intensity and complexity factor, so that a total work number was arrived at for each of the 23 procedures.

The other many procedures were evaluated by Hsiao's staff by guessing where they fell with regard to complexity. As a result of the staff's scanty experience in the eye care field, there are some bizarre rankings in which complicated reoperations for retinal detachment are ranked as less complex than the initial repair of a nondetached retina with a hole. In addition, the statisticians threw out data provided by ophthalmologists that were thought to be outliers, and those blanks were filled in with estimates of means from others, giving some real potential for bias. In addition, if an ophthalmologist did not feel comfortable in making an estimate for some procedure and left a blank, that too was filled in by the statisticians.

The researchers extrapolated and ranked the final procedures in ophthalmology. Then cross-links to other specialties were chosen. The cross-linkages to other specialties from ophthalmology are weak as there are so few procedures that we do in common with other specialties. Hsiao apparently was not convinced of the cross-linkages that were used, for the outside consultants hired by the American Academy of Ophthalmology found that the data did not check back. The researchers must have used a "fudge factor" in some fashion to assure that the ophthalmologists' relative values were on the low side. This is a serious flaw in the study and one that may cast doubt on its validity sufficient to cause many to question seriously any usefulness of the scale Hsiao has devised. This defect seems to extend to other specialties as well.

Will ophthalmologic care be affected by the Hsiao study? To answer this we should look at what will happen with the Hsiao study. At this time, the Health Care Financing Administration (HCFA) (a child of administration) and the Physician Payment Reimbursement Commission (PPRC) (a child of Congress) are both considering the study. The HCFA does not like the study because it offers no capitation system and shows little promise of reducing their expenditures, although as mentioned they may well use those procedures suggested to be overpriced to cut fees. And the PPRC, looking critically at the study, similarly sees little value in it if there is no direct advantage to Congress as it wrestles with means of reducing the budget for this year. The PPRC will probably take some of the features of the Hsiao study and come up with their own study for presentation to Congress this year. It may very well correct some of the glaring inequities in the present system of Medicare reimbursement.

If one asks, "What would the impact of the Hsiao study be if implemented close to its present recommendations?", we would simply answer, "Disruptive." Because the current Hsiao study would significantly decrease the fee structure for cataract surgery, one of the biggest governmental expenditures in the health care field and thus the single biggest income feature to the ophthalmologist, considerable adjustment of overhead and means of office practice would evolve. In fact, if the office overhead were adjusted maximally to still effect good patient care, the following are estimates of that impact by the American Academy of Ophthalmology's consultants: For those ophthalmologists who do only cataract surgery, their income would decrease by 18%; for those who do ophthalmic surgery, but no cataract surgery, their Medicare reimbursement would remain largely unchanged; and for those ophthalmologists who do no surgery, their income from Medicare would increase by 25%. One would surely interpret these figures as encouraging fewer ophthalmologists to do surgery, with the surgical load switching to fewer and fewer surgeons.

What governmental changes can be expected in implementation of a new fee structure for physicians? One would suspect that the HCFA will pay little attention to the Hsiao study except to negotiate lower fees for the physician in some manner. Congress will not want to make radical changes in medical fees, fearing both a disruption in the medical services to the aged, and a violent uprising from the strong medical lobby. Thus we can expect Congress to toy further with the fee structure, cutting fees where it can, and finding a method of implementing the PPRC's recommendations sometime in the future, using the delay to reduce the anxieties of physicians caused by rapid implementation. A factor that is rising to the surface and becoming a point of debate is the need for a national health care insurance system. For the first time in 20 years, some groups of physicians and others are saying this is what the country needs, and serious debate can be expected to mark 1989 and 1990 on the issue of national health insurance.

We can conclude that the Hsiao study will have a major impact on medical care and teaching, probably as great as that of the Flexner report many years ago. It is certainly causing a political awareness in physicians that was seldom evident in the past.

*Suggested Reading*

Editorial: Harvard RBRVS study creates controversy. *Arch Ophthalmol* 106:1516, 1988.

Frenkel M: The Resource-Based Relative Value Scale for physician compensation under Medicare: Implications for ophthalmology. *Arch Ophthalmol* 106:1669–1672, 1988.

Hsiao WC, Braun P, Yntema D, et al: Estimating physicians' work for a Resource-Based Relative Value Scale. *N Engl J Med* 319:835–841, 1988.

Hsiao WE, Braun P, Dunn D, et al: Resource-Based Relative Values: An overview. *JAMA* 260:2347–2353, 1988.

## Waveform Evolution in *Infantile* Nystagmus: An Electro-Oculo-Graphic Study of 35 Cases

Reinecke RD, Guo S, Goldstein HP (Wills Eye Hosp, Philadelphia)
*Binoc Vision* 3:191–202, Fall 1988

11–1

The definition of congenital nystagmus as nystagmus with onset at birth seems inadequate because in most patients nystagmus is not observed at birth or even within the first month of life. Congenital nystagmus has traditionally been divided into 2 types according to its waveforms, pendular and jerk; several subsets have also been identified. The true age of onset of infantile nystagmus was investigated and a more reliable calibration was documented in a series of 35 consecutive patients

### TRIANGULAR TYPE NYSTAGMUS

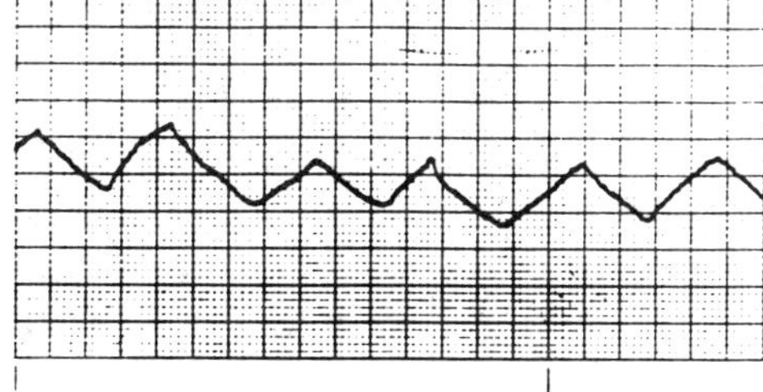

Fig 11–1.—Examples of the 3 waveforms of infantile nystagmus. (Courtesy of Reinecke RD, Guo S, Goldstein HP: *Binoc Vision* 3:191–202, Fall 1988.)

### PENDULAR TYPE NYSTAGMUS

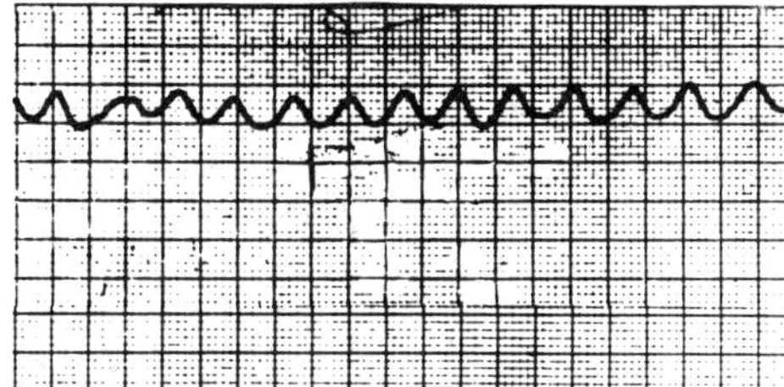

### JERK TYPE NYSTAGMUS

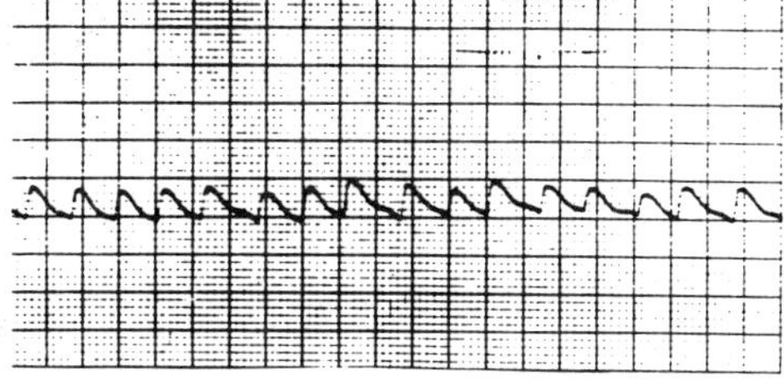

with nystagmus, only 3 of whom had nystagmus at birth or in the first 2 weeks of life.

Electrooculograms were obtained in all patients. Infantile nystagmus was found often to start with large triangular waveforms in the first to the fourth month and to evolve into smaller amplitude, higher frequency pendular waveforms that subsequently gave way to jerk waveforms within 7 months to 1½ years (Fig 11–1). Head nodding was a later common feature. The term infantile nystagmus is suggested as more appropriate for all nystagmus with onset from 1 to 8 months of age.

▶ The importance of this article lies in the recognition that the large swinging eye movements in the infant of 2–3 months typically do not represent blindness but are the first sign of infantile nystagmus. Conversely, parents of a child with a family history of nystagmus who is seen in the first month of life should not be told that nystagmus will not develop, for often it will be seen within 6 weeks or so, as described in this paper.—R.D. Reinecke, M.D.

---

**Effects of Retinal Image Stabilization in Acquired Nystagmus Due to Neurologic Disease**
Leigh RJ, Rushton DN, Thurston SE, Hertle RW, Yaniglos SS (Case Western Reserve Univ; Inst of Psychiatry, London)
*Neurology* 38:122–127, January 1988                                          11–2

---

Images must be held steadily on the retina for objects to be seen clearly and localized accurately in space. The effects of varying amounts of artificial retinal image stabilization (RIS) on oscillopsia and visual acuity were examined in 8 patients with acquired nystagmus caused by neurologic disease. Six patients had continuous oscillopsia. Horizontal and vertical eye movements were measured with the magnetic search coil method and the signals used to control the position of a visual stimulus on a screen. An optical device was used to stabilize images of the real world upon the retina (Fig 11–2).

Retinal image stabilization was progressively increased during electronic stabilization until oscillopsia was abolished. This was achieved in all eight patients and corresponded to retinal image drift of no more than 5 degrees per second. In 5 patients with downbeat nystagmus, further increases in RIS led to the reappearance of oscillopsia but in the opposite direction. Electronic stabilization improved visual acuity in 4 of 5 patients, but improvement was limited by coexisting defects in the visual system.

Artificial stabilization of images on the retina using electronic feedback is an effective means of abolishing oscillopsia in patients with neurologic nystagmus. The range of RIS required by a given individual can be measured, and from this the components of the optical device best suited for providing a stable field of vision can be calculated.

▶ Optical devices that will stabilize the images on the retina of patients with

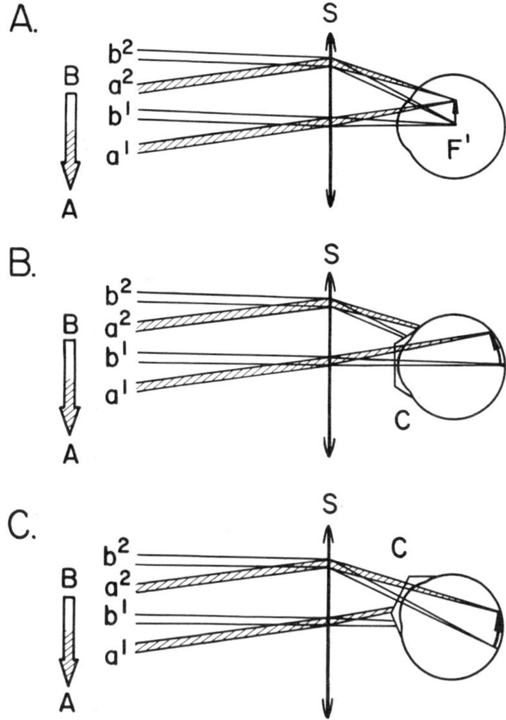



**Fig 11–2.**—An optical method for stabilizing images upon the retina. **A,** when viewing a distant object *AB,* a convergent spectacle lens, *S,* will focus rays of light *(b¹, b²)* from a point of interest *B,* on its optic axis, at its secondary focal point, *F¹,* which is close to the center of rotation of the globe. Thus if the eyeball were to rotate, light rays from point *B* would remain focused at the same point in the eye. **B,** a strongly divergent contact lens, *C,* extends back the focus from the center of the globe to the retina. **C,** because the contact lens moves with the eye, it does not negate the effect of retinal image stabilization produced by the spectacle lens, and rays of light from point *B* remain focused on the foveal region of the retina. (Courtesy of Leigh RJ, Rushton DN, Thurston SE, et al: *Neurology* 38:122–127, January 1988.)

nystagmus are becoming available. It is important for the ophthalmologic community to understand the potential for the treatment of the oscillopsia of such patients. The current paper describes a technique for finding the appropriate amount of retinal stabilization so that the oscillopsia is eliminated. Interestingly, when the object was stabilized completely, the oscillopsia reversed itself. We can expect to see such devices being used in the next few years.—R.D. Reinecke, M.D.

---

**Post-Traumatic Seesaw Nystagmus Abolished by Ethanol Ingestion**
Frisén L, Wikkelsø C (Univ of Göteborg, Göteborg, Sweden)
*Surv Ophthalmol* 32:291–292, January–February 1988                     11–3

---

Fewer than 50 reports of seesaw nystagmus have been recorded, and only 6 posttraumatic cases are known. All of these patients had severe head injury and were comatose for days or weeks. Many, and perhaps all, of the patients had extensive coexisting brain lesions, and all had bitemporal hemianopia. A late appearance of nystagmus also was characteristic; abnormal eye movements usually appeared weeks or months after head injury.

Woman, 20, experienced seesaw nystagmus and hydrocephalus several months after head trauma with resultant chiasmal injury. The nystagmus was associated with marked oscillopsia, which was markedly alleviated by ethanol consumption. A reduction in nystagmus followed the ingestion of ethanol, 1.2 gm/kg. Lumbar punctures failed to alter the nystagmus. The patient had no tendency toward alcohol abuse.

Speculation about the pathogenesis of posttraumatic seesaw nystagmus has focused on the diencephalic region. However, it may occur after brain stem stroke without chiasmal or deiencephalic lesions. The effect of ethanol on nystagmus in the described patient is not understood. A trial of propranolol might be worthwhile, because it is effective in patients with essential tremor, in whom ethanol also has a dramatic effect.

▶ Few patients have treatable nystagmus. Periodic alternating jerk nystagmus often responds to baclofen. The current article makes the unique contribution that the oral intake of alcohol reduced seesaw nystagmus. Further, the patient was seen to have a continuing reduction in the nystagmus after taking clonazepam orally. Only by the careful observations of such unique responses do we have hope that the true mechanism of nystagmus in man may be understood and appropriate treatment evolved.—R.D. Reinecke, M.D.

---

## A Single Dominant Gene Can Account for Eye Tracking Dysfunctions and Schizophrenia in Offspring of Discordant Twins

Holzman PS, Kringlen E, Matthysse S, Flanagan SD, Lipton RB, Cramer G, Levin S, Lange K, Levy DL (Harvard Univ, Cambridge; Harvard Med School, Boston; McLean Hosp, Belmont, Mass; Univ of Oslo, Beckman Research Inst of the City of Hope, Duarte, Calif; et al)
*Arch Gen Psychiatry* 45:641–647, July 1988                    11–4

---

Eye movement dysfunctions (EMDs), which are detectable in smooth pursuit, occur in most patients with schizophrenia and in 45% of their first-degree relatives. Previous research suggests that these EMDs represent a biologic marker for schizophrenia. The mode of transmission of the schizophrenia-EMD complex was studied by recording the eye movements of offspring of monozygotic and dizygotic twins. Twins were selected if 1 twin met the criteria for schizophrenia, bipolar affective disorder, or reactive psychosis.

The series included 214 patients. It was determined that EMDs and at least some schizophrenias can be considered expressons of a single underlying trait transmitted by an autosomal dominant gene.

▶ This article is fascinating. When schizophrenia and EMD of saccadic intrusions and macrosquare waves during pursuit eye movements are considered together, they are inherited as a dominant autosomal trait. Ophthalmologists can be expected to know of this condition and to offer interpretation of the smooth pursuit abnormalities. Although not covered in this paper, the abnormalities of the eye movements cited here have not been established as being clinically significant in actual visual performance.—R.D. Reinecke, M.D.

## Eye Movement Abnormalities as a Predictor of the Acquired Immunodeficiency Syndrome Dementia Complex

Currie J, Benson E, Ramsden B, Perdices M, Cooper D (Mental Health Research Inst of Victoria, Melbourne; Monash Univ Med School, Victoria; Univ of New South Wales, Sydney)
*Arch Neurol* 45:949–953, September 1988                    11–5

In attempting to establish an early diagnosis of acquired immunodeficiency syndrome (AIDS)–dementia complex (ADC), studies have shown abnormalities in detailed neuropsychometric testing in patients with AIDS who have apparently normal findings on routine neurologic and mental state testing. Because eye movements can be controlled, recorded, and quantified with greater precision than most other interactive physiologic parameters, they are an excellent means of probing brain function in disorders of higher cortical function. Whether the severity of dementia could be correlated with abnormalities of eye movement, and whether eye movement abnormalities could be detected before onset of clinical dementia, were determined in a group of patients with AIDS, with or without ADC, using infrared oculography.

Eye movement abnormalities were noted in all 7 patients with mild, moderate, or severe ADC and in 6 of 7 with AIDS or human immunodeficiency virus (HIV) antibodies without clinical dementia but at risk for ADC. These abnormalities included disturbances in both saccadic and smooth-pursuit function, and their severity correlated strongly with the severity of dementia. The abnormalities were qualitatively similar to those occurring in Alzheimer's disease but quantitatively less severe.

Recording eye movements may be a valuable noninvasive method for early detection of neurologic dysfunction in asymptomatic patients who test positive for HIV or in patients with AIDS, even before other clinical evidence of ADC is available. This approach may be particularly useful in identifying high-risk patients who require antiviral therapy and in monitoring the neurologic response to such therapy.

▶ With the increasing prevalence of AIDS, it is common to see such patients in many hospitals. I found it of considerable interest that AIDS patients have eye movement disorders similar to those in patients with Alzheimer's disease. Because these abnormalities are often a precursor to the severe dementia of AIDS, it is well to be aware of this relationship. I suspect more work will have to be done to confirm the results of this important study.—R.D. Reinecke, M.D.

---

## Treatment of Acquired Nystagmus With Botulinum A Toxin

Helveston EM, Pogrebniak AE (Indiana Univ, Indianapolis)
*Am J Ophthalmol* 106:584–586, November 1988                    11–6

Botulinum A toxin is used to treat certain types of nystagmus, blepharospasm, and Meige's disease. The toxin was used to treat vertical, horizontal, and rotary pendular nystagmus after brain stem stroke that produced oscillopsia in 2 patients. Botulinum A toxin was injected into the retrobulbar space of 1 eye in each patient. Acuity improved from 20/80 to 20/30 in 1 patient, and both were able to read and watch television after treatment. Visual improvement lasted for 5–13 weeks. Five injections of 25 units in each patient caused no adverse side effects.

Toxin injection in these eyes probably produced paresis of all of the extraocular muscles, leading to reduced ocular movement and subjective improvement in oscillopsia. In both cases sedentary activities such as watching television were important. The dose used is well below that causing systemic toxicity. Repeat injections are required, but this approach is useful in patients with acquired nystagmus that impairs vision to a disabling degree.

---

## Changes in Astigmatism Between the Ages of 1 and 4 Years: A Longitudinal Study

Abrahamsson M, Fabian G, Sjöstrand J (Univ of Göteborg; Västerås, Sweden)
*Br J Ophthalmol* 72:145–149, 1988                    11–7

A 4-year follow-up was made of a population sample of 299 astigmatic infants to document developmental changes in astigmatism. The cycloplegic refraction was monitored annually in consecutive infants aged 1 year with astigmatism of 1.0 D or more in at least 1 eye.

The degree of hypermetropia did not decrease during development, but the incidence and amount of astigmatism decreased significantly. The most marked decline in astigmatism occurred in the second year of life. Most astigmatic eyes initially had a horizontal curvature greater than the vertical, and no change in the axis of astigmatism was observed during follow-up.

These findings confirm a decrease in astigmatism as infants grow older, particularly between the first and second years of life. Patients having with-the-rule or oblique astigmatism at age 1 year require special follow-up.

▶ Much has been made of the finding of rather large amounts of astigmatism in the neonate. This paper is important to place the reduction of astigmatism in perspective, yet calls attention to the necessity of carefully following those infants with oblique astigmatism and with-the-rule astigmatism. The ophthalmologist is probably on safe grounds in not prescribing astigmatic corrections in the young child unless the astigmatism is more than 2 D or asymmetric.—R.D. Reinecke, M.D.

## Morning-to-Evening Change in Refraction, Corneal Curvature, and Visual Acuity 2 to 4 Years After Radial Keratotomy in the PERK Study

Santos VR, Waring GO III, Lynn MJ, Schanzlin DJ, Cantillo N, Espinal ME, Garbus J, Justin N, Roszka-Duggan V (PERK Coordinating Ctrs, Emory Univ)
*Ophthalmology* 95:1487–1493, November 1988                    11–8

Fifty-two patients in whom ophthalmic measurements were made at 3 months and 1 year in the Prospective Evaluation of Radial Keratotomy (PERK) study of radial keratotomy were again evaluated 2½ to 4 years postoperatively. Measurements were made before 10 A.M. and after 5:30 P.M. on the same day.

Thirty-one percent of eyes had an increase in minus spherical equivalent power of the manifest refraction of 0.5–1.5 D between the 2 examinations (Fig 11–3). Another 12% had a change in cylinder power of 0.5–1.0 D, and 19% had a decrease in uncorrected acuity of 2–5

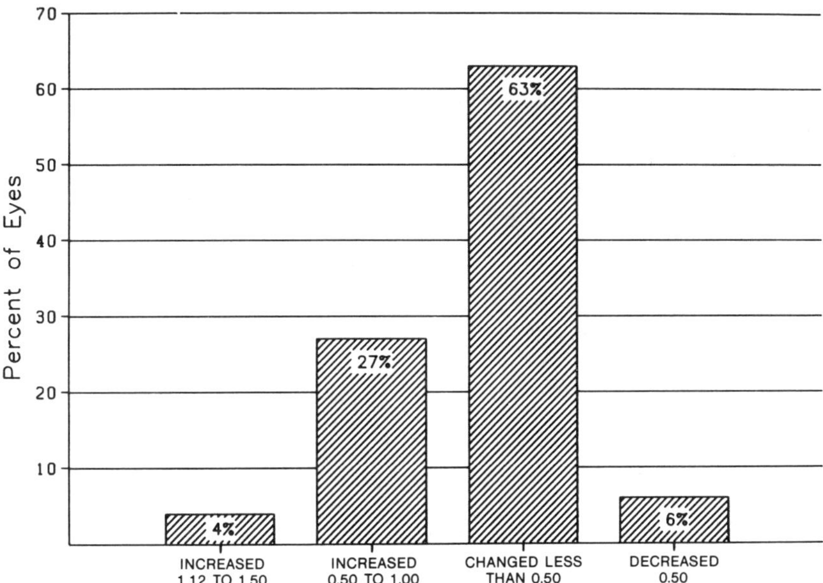


Change in Minus Power of the Manifest Refraction (D)
from Morning to Evening at 3.5 Years

Fig 11–3.—The change from morning to evening in the manifest refraction *(D)* measured at 2–4 years after surgery. The *bar height* indicates the percent of eyes with each change in the manifest refraction. (Courtesy of Santos VR, Waring GO III, Lynn MJ, et al: *Ophthalmology* 95:1487–1493, November 1988.)

Snellen lines. Overall, 29% of the eyes had central corneal steepening by 0.5–1.0 D.

Morning-to-evening fluctuation in refraction can persist for several years after radial keratotomy. However, the visual changes in the present patients are not necessarily representative of the PERK population. Slow corneal wound healing may be a major factor in the refractive change. It can take as long as 5 years for unsutured keratotomy wounds to heal, and remodeling of the wounds also takes many years. It is not clear whether the postkeratotomy cornea has as stable a shape as the normal cornea once wound healing is complete. Possible factors in changing corneal shape include corneal edema beneath the closed lid, early morning elevation in intraocular pressure, and mechanical pressure of the closed lid on the cornea.

## Monocular Diplopia Accompanying Ordinary Refractive Errors

Coffeen P, Guyton DL (Johns Hopkins Univ)
*Am J Ophthalmol* 105:451–459, May 1988                                 11–9

Many individuals normally can experience monocular diplopia under certain conditions, such as irregular refraction or decentered contact lenses. Neurologic causes of monocular diplopia are rare. Trial lenses were used to induce varying spherical refractive errors in 11 eyes of 9 persons who viewed radial patterns of lines under dim room illumination.

All 9 reported doubling in at least 1 defocused condition. The doubling consistently disappeared when a pinhole aperture was introduced. Radially symmetric doubling occurred in 1 of 11 eyes with induced myopia and in 3 eyes with induced hyperopia. Defocusing the astigmatic dial pattern on the screen produced blurring but not doubling.

Refractive error should not be overlooked as contributing to monocular diplopia. It is a frequent and readily correctable cause. If refractive error is corrected early in the evaluation of a patient who complains of monocular diplopia, more extensive studies may not be necessary.

▶ Monocular diplopia is often ignored or leads to unnecessary work-ups. The authors have given us some good hints to avoid mistakes. In addition to their suggestions I would add that one should look for chalazions and the like, which create just enough astigmatism to cause certain individuals to experience diplopia, particularly at night as the pupil dilates. Amateur astronomers are particularly sensitive to such monocular diplopia.—R.D. Reinecke, M.D.

## Refraction Problems After Refractive Surgery

Rowsey JJ, Rubin ML (Univ of Oklahoma; Univ of Florida)
*Surv Ophthalmol* 32:414–420, May–June 1988                          11–10

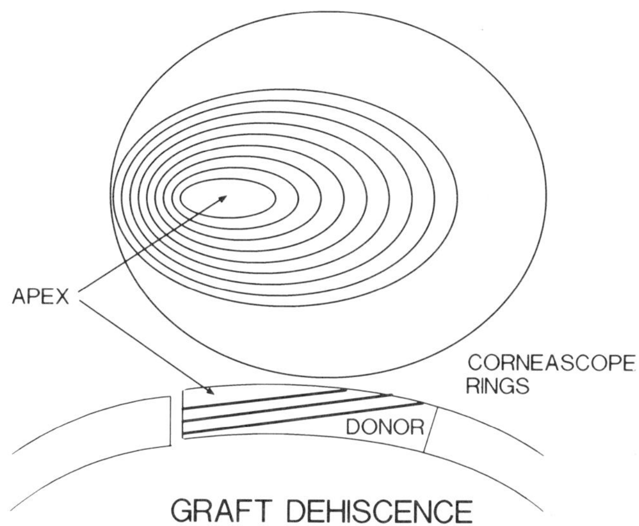


**Fig 11–4.**—Corneal graft after suture removal. The graft edge has slipped forward. Diagram of the corneascope rings shows them centered on the high point (apex) of the anteriorly displaced edge. The ring pattern shows the marked astigmatism that has been generated. (Courtesy of Rowsey JJ, Rubin ML: *Surv Ophthalmol* 32:414–420, May–June 1988.)

Several surgical procedures now are used to alter the corneal power by modifying the central or peripheral corneal topography. In refracting a patient after radial keratotomy, it is helpful to use a dimly lit room and to "crowd" as much plus power as is accepted without blurring distance vision. That refraction then is over-minused by 0.5 D to compensate in part for the induced myopia accompanying pupillary dilation. If vision fluctuates substantially during the day, cycloplegic refraction is done in both the morning and late afternoon. Rarely, a patient will require 2 sets of glasses. If the patient is an early presbyope, postoperative problems should be expected.

New methods of monitoring corneal curvature will be useful for following patients after refractive surgery. Contact lens fitting after refractive surgery is problematic, but it succeeds occasionally. If astigmatism is present after operation, careful study of the retinoscopic pattern or Placido disk photokeratoscopy probably will show the cause of the problem. If 1 edge of the graft is shifted forward and coreneascope rings are markedly decentered (Fig 11–4), the wound must be resutured. Any surgery for astigmatism can radically change the existing refraction. Undercorrection is preferable to overcorrection, as in most other types of surgery.

▶ Refractive surgery is being performed on more and more patients. These patients eventually come to see any ophthalmologist for second opinions and checkups. Thus this article is particularly timely. I concur with giving the young patient the additional minus, but care must be taken in doing so with the patient older than 30 years of age, as they are usually happier with the full plus.

An AM appointment should be given the first time a new patient of this type is seen, as any corneal edema will be more apparent. The next visit should be in the late PM to look for the daily refractive changes.—R.D. Reinecke, M.D.

## Developmental Aspects of the Brückner Test
Archer SM (Indiana Univ, Indianapolis)
*Ophthalmology* 95:1098–1101, August 1988                                    11–11

Examination of the fundus reflexes is potentially of greatest value in assessing the youngest infants and children for strabismus and amblyopia. Such examination provides information about the status of binocular function that cannot be obtained by usual means. However, little attention has been given to age-related variations in the fundus reflex phenomena observed during Brückner testing. The development of fundus reflex phenomena was investigated in 1,342 examinations performed in normal infants, ranging in age from newborn to 10 months.

In most infants who were at least 8 months of age, characteristic symmetric dimming of the fundus reflexes in both eyes occurred with central fixation. Neonates and most infants younger than 2 months did not have dimming of the fundus reflex with fixation, probably because of inability to accommodate accurately. From 2 to 8 months of age, up to 28% of the infants had asymmetric dimming of the fundus reflexes in both eyes. Unlike older children, in whom this is a pathologic finding, asymmetric fundus reflexes in children in this age group may represent a normal stage of development.

Infants aged 2–8 months have an unacceptably high frequency of positive findings on the Brückner test, but only a small fraction of these are likely to be associated with any permanent abnormalities. The fundus reflex phenomena observed in the course of performing the Brückner test should thus not be used for screening in infants younger than 8 months.

▶ The Brückner test is quick and easy to use. It simply measures the equality of the red reflex when a patient looks at the ophthalmoscope at 0.5 m. If the color is equal, the eyes are aligned; if not, the lighter reflex indicates the deviated eye. Archer has pointed out that the Brückner test should not be used as a screening test in children younger than 8 months—an important point.—R.D. Reinecke, M.D.

## Visual Acuity, Strabismus, and Amblyopia in Premature Babies With and Without Retinopathy of Prematurity
Snir M, Nissenkorn I, Sherf I, Cohen S, Sira IB (Beilinson Med Ctr, Petach Tikva; Tel Aviv Univ, Israel)
*Ann Ophthalmol* 20:256–258, July 1988                                    11–12

The increasing survival rate of premature infants weighing less than 1,500 gm is accompanied by anatomical and functional ocular complications caused by the increased incidence of retinopathy of prematurity

(ROP). The incidence of refractive errors, strabismus, and amblyopia with and without cicatricial ROP was investigated in 187 premature infants born between 1973 and 1981. Of these, 48 had ROP.

The incidence of strabismus in the group with cicatricial ROP was 23%, compared with 9% in the group without cicatricial ROP. Amblyopia was noted in 6% of the group with ROP and in only 1.4% of those without it. Myopia occurred in 50% of the infants with ROP and in 15% of those without ROP. Astigmatism and anisometropia were also more common among infants with ROP, but hypermetropia was represented equally in both groups.

▶ The famous answer of Willy Sutton to "Why do you rob banks?" was "Because that's where the money is." This certainly applies to the examination of an infant whose birth weight is 1,500 gm or less. These low-birth-weight babies need not only a complete examination to rule out ROP, but both those with and those without ROP need to be observed carefully. I like to see them at least once a year, because they are the children who, as this article notes, have significant refractive errors, strabismus, and amblyopia.—R.D. Reinecke, M.D.

---

**Hospitalization Requirements After Vitreoretinal Surgery**
Isernhagen RD, Michels RG, Glaser BM, de Bustros S, Enger C (Johns Hopkins Univ)
*Arch Ophthalmol* 106:767–770, June 1988                     11–13

---

Hospitalization needs were determined in 200 patients having vitreoretinal surgery. Half of the patients had postoperative events best managed in a hospital setting. Forty-four patients had pain necessitating intramuscular injections 5 hours or more after surgery. Thirty-five patients required medication intramuscularly because of nausea. Thirty patients required physician consultation for medical illness 5 or more hours after surgery. Forty-one patients required more than 1 postoperative day of hospitalization because of ocular abnormalities.

Half of the patients in this prospective study had indications for inpatient treatment after vitreoretinal surgery. Most had retinal detachment or complications of proliferative diabetic retinopathy. Patients having surgery on the same eye in the preceding 2 months and those younger than 30 years of age were especially likely to require inpatient care. Other factors were a diagnosis of proliferative vitreoretinopathy or penetrating ocular injury, vitrectomy with scleral buckling or silicone oil injection, and surgery lasting for more than 1 hour. Most patients having vitreoretinal surgery require hospitalization for optimal care.

---

**Prevalence of Illegal Motor Vehicle Driving Among Visually Impaired Elderly Patients in Alberta**
Paetkau ME, Taerum T, Hiebert T (Univ of Alberta, Edmonton)
*Can J Ophthalmol* 23:301–304, December 1988                     11–14

---

Best Corrected Visual Acuity Among the Patients
Who Were Driving Illegally

| Acuity | | No. (and %) of patients |
| --- | --- | --- |
| Poorer eye | Better eye | (n = 22) |
| Counting fingers | Counting fingers | 1  (4) |
| 6/120 | 6/120 | 3 (14) |
| 6/60–counting fingers | 6/60 | 4 (18) |
| 6/60–counting fingers | 6/30 | 5 (23) |
| 6/24–counting fingers | 6/18–6/24 | 6 (27) |
| 6/21–hand movements | 6/12 | 3 (14) |

(Courtesy of Paetkau ME, Taerum T, Hiebert T: *Can J Ophthalmol* 23:301–304, December 1988.)

Among nearly 500 patients aged 65 and older who were referred consecutively to a sight enhancement clinic in northern Alberta, 22 (4%) with vision less than the legal limit persisted in driving a motor vehicle (table). Men were more likely than women to drive with inadequate vision. Of the 21 patients driving legally, 11 were legally blind in 1 eye. Sixteen of the 22 patients driving illegally had age-related maculopathy and 3 had nonproliferative diabetic retinopathy. Nearly all of the patients had disorders associated with large permanent paracentral scotomas. One patient each had inoperable cellophane maculopathy, amblyopia plus central retinal artery occlusion, and optic nerve disease.

Several of these persons drove despite being eligible to register with the Canadian National Institute for the Blind. Three diabetics who required insulin injections drove illegally. None of these patients were reported by their physicians as not being able to drive safely. It should not be assumed that all legally blind persons seek visual help or that physicians reliably report them to the authorities. Physicians' responsibilities include taking measures that can prevent motor vehicle accidents.

## Advertising in Ophthalmology

Margo CE, Trobe JD, Lowenstein JH, Slamovits TL (Univ of South Florida, Tampa; Univ of Michigan; Albert Einstein College of Medicine, Bronx)
*Surv Ophthalmol* 33:211–216, November–December 1988                    11–15

*Part I. Advertising Is a Threat to Professional Autonomy*
Advertising for ophthalmologic services is increasingly reliant on marketing methods usually reserved for nonmedical services. Commercial advertising can, by its very nature, mislead, and some types of medical advertising are actually detrimental to the public and the profession. There is little objective reason to conclude that advertising leads to inferior care, or injures patients, or results in unnecessary surgery. It also is difficult to demonstrate that medical advertising lowers medical costs through increased competition. The real risk is that of losing professional credibility. Only a minority of ophthalmologists advertise, but their actions influence the entire profession.—C.E. Margo, M.D.

*Part II. Advertising Is a Defensible Aspect of Free Enterprise*
Possibly one fourth of ophthalmic practices now advertise on television. Such advertising is believed to be helpful because it makes more information and choices available. Patients are harmed more by incompetent practice than by false advertising. Those opposed to advertising contend that patients cannot protect themselves from being duped because medicine is so complicated and illness often precludes rationality. These considerations suggest that patients be given more rather than less information.—J.D. Trobe, M.D.; J.H. Lowenstein, J.D.

*Part III. Editorial*
Advertising is a reality, and the best that can be hoped for is that it be as free as possible of misinformation, deception, misleading claims, and unprofessional conduct. Both self-policing and prompt notification of potential violations of the Academy's ethical code are important.—T.L. Slamovits, M.D.

# Subject Index

## L

## S

# Author Index